The Apple Cider Vinegar Cleanse

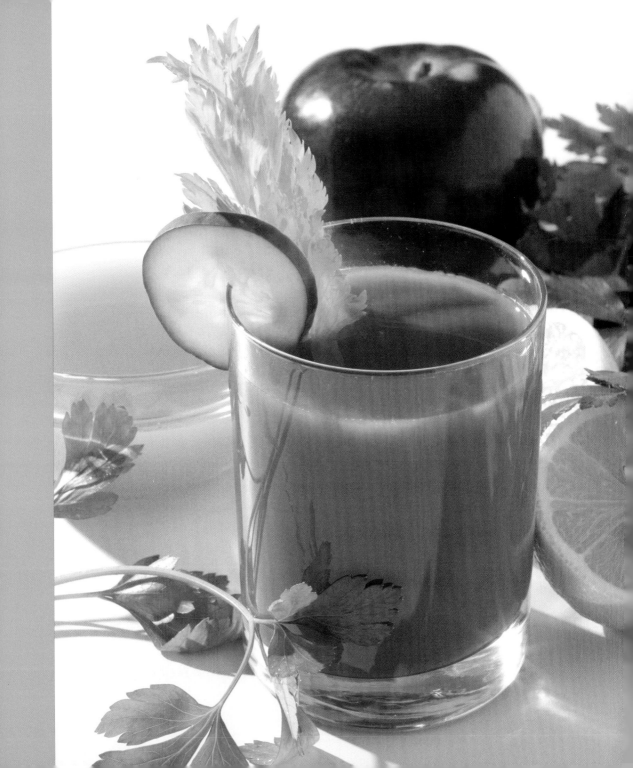

The Apple Cider Vinegar Cleanse

Lose Weight, Improve Gut Health, Fight Cholesterol,
and More with Nature's Miracle Cure

CLAIRE **GEORGIOU**,
B.HSC (C.MED) ND MATMS

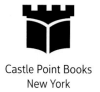

Castle Point Books
New York

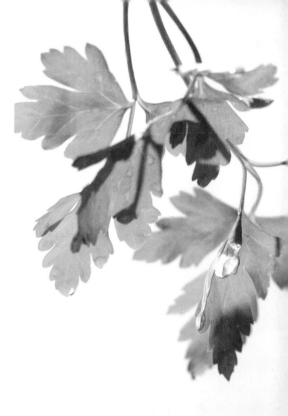

Acknowledgments

I want to thank my family and friends for always listening to me babble about health continually over the many years, my patients for always kindly sharing their journey with me. Thanks also to all of the amazing people that I have had the pleasure of working with who have continually supported me in learning as much as I can, to all the people in the natural health community who have continued to inspire me to work toward a health change for all.

And I most importantly want to thank my husband, family and my children for bearing with me while I busily wrote this book. I am grateful for their patience, and for helping me taste test all of the recipes to ensure that they were as tasty as they were nutritious and healthy.

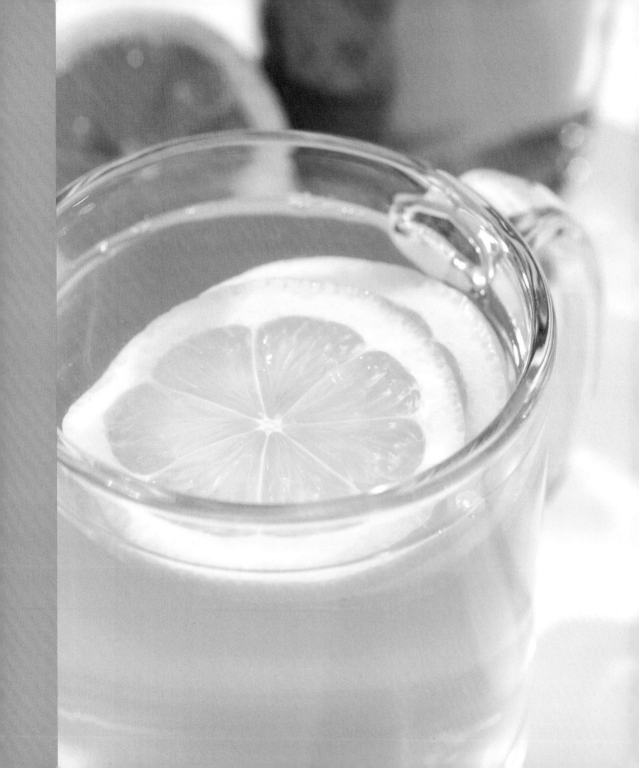

Contents

chapter 2. What Is the ACV Cleanse?

chapter 4. Sticking to Your ACV Cleanse

Introduction

Good health is the cornerstone of a happy, enjoyable life. With so many environmental influences and lifestyle factors, it can be hard to manage your life to reach the level of health you deserve.

I wanted to write this book to share some of the knowledge I have accumulated in the many years of practicing as a naturopath and nutritionist using nutritional therapy, superfoods, plant-based recipes, and health protocols that I know work!

I have spent many years working with the Reboot team for Joe Cross, supporting people who are partaking in juice fasts and other programs. The number of health changes I have witnessed working in a clinic with Dr. Sandra Cabot and the Reboot team has been remarkable. In this book, I have included many tips and tricks that I learned as a practitioner.

This book is designed to help you achieve a healthier version of yourself, whether that means shedding those unwanted pounds, supporting a healthier immune system, improving your gut health, reducing the occurrence of allergies, increasing stamina and energy, or just improving your general well-being.

Natural foods and plants have so many beneficial ingredients, and they're packed with compounds and naturally occurring phytonutrients that support a healthy body, both physically and mentally. I am truly passionate about good health and its ability to help you live your best life possible, a life that is filled with ample energy and disease prevention.

It is estimated that 70% of all chronic disease is preventable with daily healthy lifestyle practices, including a healthy diet. It always saddens me to see so many people living with chronic health conditions that can be reversed with time, practice, healthy eating, and some self-love. I want to empower those who can make the changes to do so, so they can enjoy a rich, healthy, and fulfilling life.

Combining the benefits of juicing, consuming more fruits and vegetables, and a healthy dose of ACV is a perfect way to jumpstart a healthy lifestyle. This diet not only will increase your nutrient intake, but also will provide the best environment for your body to support its natural detoxification pathways and allow many positive health changes to occur.

Remember this plan is a jumping off platform to encourage healthier eating on a long-term basis. By following the plan, you will be able to moderate your hunger and gain the health you deserve.

This combines some very important cleansing protocols that will help balance your blood sugar levels, increase your metabolism rate, maintain healthy bowel ecology, improve liver health, improve detoxification functions, reset your hormones, and reduce the risk of many chronic health conditions and diseases.

I would also like to clearly state that this is NOT a fad diet, but rather a fantastic starting point for practicing healthier eating patterns, learning new kitchen skills, and avoiding all addictive processed foods. On this plan, you will only eat clean and plant-based foods for 7 days.

It truly is a cleansing diet. This diet is 100% free of all processed foods; you will eat only plant-based foods, with the addition of fat-burning drinks to support your health changes.

This plan will jump-start hormonal changes that shift your metabolism from fat-making to fat-burning! This shift can take a few days to begin after your water weight is lost and your appetite regulation is achieved. By day 3, your body will go straight into a fat-burning state, and your appetite will be reduced.

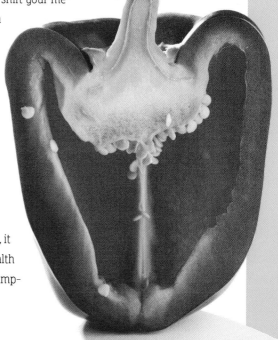

By avoiding all processed foods, sugar, and alcohol, you can allow your body to eliminate those food and beverage addictions and move on to healthier long-term eating. All food on the plan is light, easy on the digestive system, and packed with nutrients.

It is important to note that apple cider vinegar may not work for everyone in every way listed. Overall, it will provide many health benefits and support good health and well-being. This book is dedicated to helping you jump-start your health in preparation for a healthier lifestyle!

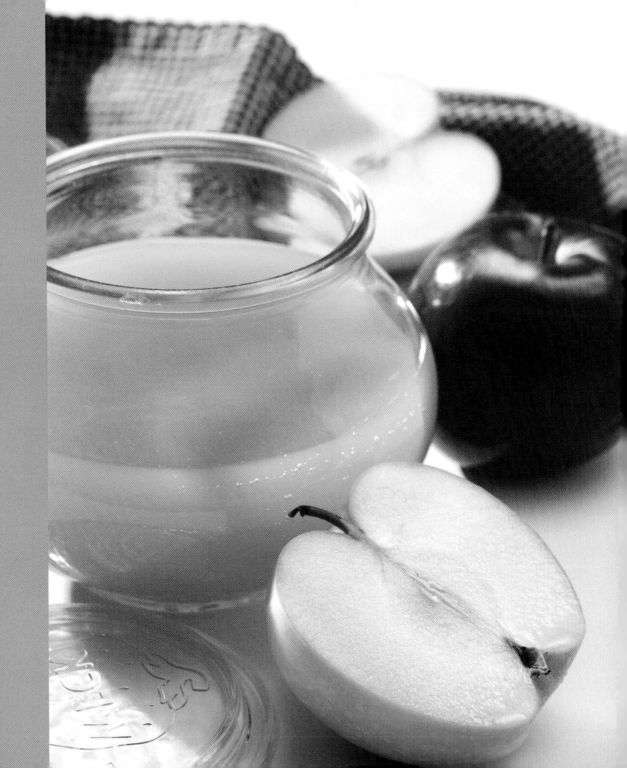

chapter 1. **What** Is **Apple Cider** Vinegar?

Apple cider vinegar has been used for thousands of years for everything from healing wounds to treating blood sugar irregularities and polishing furniture. Many people around the world have considered apple cider vinegar a cure-all product, and it can support your health in so many ways. Apple cider vinegar is inexpensive, easy to find, and has a multitude of uses. Apple cider vinegar is also known as cider vinegar or ACV.

Apple cider vinegar is made by crushing fresh apples and allowing them to mature in barrels with added yeast. They then ferment into alcohol. Bacteria are added to convert the alcohol into vinegar for the second stage of fermentation. When the vinegar is mature, it will contain a dark, cloudy, weblike bacterial foam called "mother," which becomes visible when the rich brownish liquid is held to the light.

The only ACV I recommend is the **unpasteurized organic apple cider vinegar** that still contains the mother tincture, rather than the filtered processed vinegars you may see in supermarkets. The mother is a very special ingredient, which includes living nutrients and friendly bacteria. The mother is also known as *Mycoderma aceti*. Mother of vinegar is created when acetic acid bacteria and a type of cellulose develop during the fermentation process.

I also highly recommend purchasing ACV in glass containers due to the acetic acid, which has a lower pH and can be corrosive to any unstable plastic chemicals and solvents (including BPA and BPS) present in plastic containers.

Other inherent bioactive components of ACV include gallic acid, catechin, epicatechin, chlorogenic acid, caffeic acid, and *p*-coumaric acid. These ACV compounds contain antioxidative, antidiabetic, antimicrobial, antitumor, anti-obesity, and antihypertensive properties. They can also help lower your cholesterol.

The History of Vinegar

The earliest known use of vinegar was 10,000 years ago. The Babylonians made many types of vinegars that were flavored with fruits, honey, and malts. The Roman Army, once the most powerful and formidable conquerors of the known world, used an ACV tonic to stay strong and healthy.

There are references in the Old Testament and from Hippocrates where vinegar was used as a natural antibiotic, antiseptic, and wound healer. In China around the 10th century, vinegar was used as an antiseptic hand wash to prevent infection. Early U.S. medical practitioners used vinegar to treat croup, stomachache, fever, and edema.

ACV Health Benefits and Uses

Curative apple cider vinegar has been an age-old home remedy to ease health ailments and restore the body. Modern studies are now finding that these anecdotes are not just coincidence, but truly effective!

HEALTHY BLOOD SUGAR LEVELS

Unstable blood sugar will negatively impact your health, energy, and weight loss, along with a range of chronic inflammatory diseases. People who suffer from hypoglycemia, insulin resistance, and diabetes all have an impaired ability to maintain stable blood sugar levels due to impaired cell sensitivity to insulin and sugar.

Studies have found that vinegar may help to lower glucose levels, making it a beneficial treatment for people with hypoglycemia, insulin resistance, and type 2 diabetes. A 2007 study from Arizona State University found that taking two tablespoons of apple cider vinegar along with a small portion of food before going to sleep led to a 4–6 % decrease in fasting blood sugar levels. They then fed the group a high-carbohydrate breakfast and saw less sugar spikes in the ACV control group. The antiglycemic effect of acetic acid, the active ingredient in vinegar, has been attributed to reduced starch digestion and delayed gastric emptying, which influences the glycemic effect of carbohydrate-based meals. This also has the benefit of supporting appetite regulation, cravings, and weight loss.

This particular study didn't show a huge drop, but it's a great indication of the effect ACV can have on a long-term basis with the addition of a healthy and balanced diet.

In another study, vinegar was shown to improve insulin sensitivity from a high-carb meal by 19–34% and significantly lower blood glucose and insulin responses. Insulin sensitivity has been improved through vinegar treatment in 19% of individuals with type 2 diabetes and 34% of individuals with pre-diabetes. This is big news in terms of the effect ACV can have on improving insulin sensitivity, which in turn means the need for less insulin production. This has a significant effect on insulin resistance, weight loss, and possibly diabetic control.

Another study performed performed by the Applied Nutrition and Food Chemistry division at Lund University in Sweden found that consuming vinegar with a high carbohydrate potato-based meal significantly reduced the post-meal sugar spike. Therefore, the results showed that the high glycemic and insulinemic features commonly associated with high-carbohydrate meals can be reduced by the use of vinegar dressing or simply by sipping on ACV mixed with water.

In 2010, Arizona State University published a study examining the effects of acetic acid on post-meal glucose levels. The study found that when people consume small doses of vinegar *during* meals that consist of complex carbohydrates, instead of taking it several hours prior, the vinegar effectively reduced post-meal glycemia by 20% more than the placebo.

Research published in the *European Journal of Clinical Nutrition* found that the post-meal glycemic decrease was dependent on the dose of vinegar. In the study, increased doses of vinegar lead to reduced blood glucose and insulin responses, while increasing the participants' likelihood of feeling full. So, the higher the intake of vinegar, the better the blood sugar levels, and the better the appetite satiety. So, drink up!

WEIGHT LOSS

Given that vinegar lowers blood sugar and insulin levels, it makes sense that it could also help you lose weight. Weight problems are on the rise. In fact, more than 30% of U.S. citizens are classified as obese, and another 30% are overweight.

Several studies suggest that vinegar can increase satiety, helping you eat fewer calories and lose weight. It is estimated that when people consume vinegar with their meals they are likely to consume 200–275 fewer calories per day.

Apple cider vinegar has been shown to regulate the glycemic index of foods by slowing down the digestion of the sugars. The acetic acid found in vinegar helps to regulate the speed at which the sugar absorbs into the intestines; this then causes a reduction in any possible sugar spikes, which helps to reduce insulin and appetite spikes.

A 2005 Swedish study found that people felt fuller and more satisfied for longer periods of time after eating bread with vinegar, as opposed to eating bread on its own.

One small Japanese study published in 2009 in the *Journal of Bioscience, Biotechnology and Biochemistry* studied the effects of consuming 15 mL or 30 mL of acetic acid (the major component of vinegar) diluted in water every day for twelve weeks.

The results were as follows:

A study in obese individuals showed that daily vinegar consumption led to reduced belly fat, waist circumference, lower blood triglycerides, and weight loss:

- 15 mL (1 tablespoon): Lost 2.6 pounds (1.2 kilograms)
- 30 mL (2 tablespoons): Lost 3.7 pounds (1.7 kilograms)

A 2009 study from the *Journal of Agricultural and Food Chemistry* found that when mice were fed a high-fat diet and given acetic acid (found in vinegar) they developed 10 percent less body fat (as compared to mice that were not given acetic acid). The study's authors suggest that acetic acid may prevent the build-up of body fat by activating genes involved in breaking down fats.

CHOLESTEROL

There are two main types of cholesterol: LDL (which is often called "bad cholesterol") and HDL (which is often called "good cholesterol"). LDL cholesterol encourages fat in the bloodstream, while HDL cholesterol removes excess LDL cholesterol and triglycerides from the bloodstream, thus protecting our cardiovascular health. The higher the LDL to HDL ratio, the higher the risk for the development of heart disease will be.

A 2012 study published in *Life Science Journal* revealed that consumption of apple cider vinegar over an eight-week period could significantly reduce blood lipids that contribute to high cholesterol and triglyceride levels in people who suffer from hyperlipidemia (high levels of fat in the blood).

In an animal-based study published in the *Pakistan Journal of Biological Sciences*, scientists found that diabetic rats that were fed an apple-cider-vinegar-enhanced diet for four weeks experienced an increase in HDL cholesterol, as well as a reduction in triglycerides.

Furthermore, apple cider vinegar contains high levels of polyphenols such chlorogenic acid. These polyphenols were linked to the prevention of cardiovascular diseases, improved health, and the inhibition of LDL oxidation.

HYPERTENSION

When blood pressure stays elevated for long periods of time, it can increase the risk of heart disease and stroke.

According to a study in *Bioscience, Biotechnology, and Biochemistry*, when rats consumed apple cider vinegar, they had reductions in blood pressure levels. It was determined that the reduction in blood pressure was due to the acetic acid in apple cider vinegar.

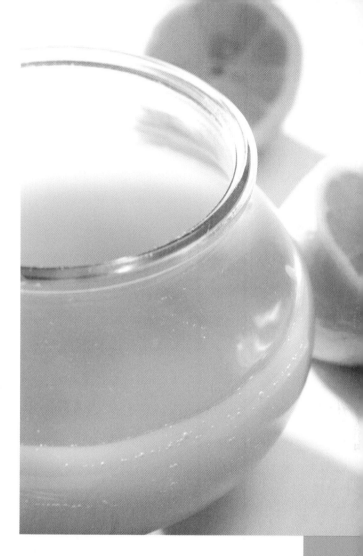

ANTI-CANCER BENEFITS

Most of the studies on the correlation between vinegar and cancer cells have been performed in test tubes and in animal studies. In studies involving rats and mice, rice vinegar extracts were shown to be protective against colon cancer.

Kurosu vinegar has also been found to inhibit the growth of a variety of cancerous cells, including those of the lung, breast, bladder, and prostate.

Kibizu, a Japanese sugar cane vinegar, has been shown in cell studies to inhibit the growth of leukemia cells. Consuming vinegar may even reduce the risk of esophageal cancer. This is not ACV, but it gives us some very insightful information into how vinegar can really impact and change our health for the better.

ARTHRITIS

Arthritis is a very common disability. Arthritis includes inflammation of the joints and surrounding tissues; certain types of arthritis may also involve the immune system.

I repeatedly heard about consuming ACV for arthritis while I was working in a natural foods store when I was young. So many happy elderly people swore by it. It was my first introduction to the magical properties of apple cider vinegar. And yes, it's now backed by science for a variety of health problems. But many people have been enjoying the benefits of ACV for centuries. There are reports that it can alleviate symptoms within only 1–2 weeks.

For pain, mix 1 tablespoon ACV into warm water. If you'd like, add 1 teaspoon of honey. This concoction can greatly reduce pain and increase mobility.

DETOXIFICATION SUPPORT

The naturally occurring phenolic compounds have a supportive role in reducing oxidative stress and inflammation along with stimulating efficient bile production, which is how the body supports the removal of waste and unhealthy fats.

GALLBLADDER HEALTH

I recommend apple cider vinegar to help reduce gallbladder discomfort and improve gallbladder emptying. If you have gallstones, it is very important that you start introducing ACV into your diet. Slowly increase your consumption until you are comfortably including the average recommended dose.

INFECTIONS

Because acetic acid kills unwanted bacteria when it comes into contact with it, it essentially acts as a natural antibiotic and antiseptic. ACV has traditionally been used for warts, nail fungal infections, ear infections, gut infections, throat infections, skin infections, and more. Thousands of years ago, Hippocrates, the father of medicine, used it as a wound cleanser.

GUT MICROBIOME

ACV has been shown to kill unhealthy bacteria and other microbes in the digestive tract, such as Candida. It is also known to promote the production of healthy bacteria.

Due to the pectin content, it can help soothe and support an upset stomach and provide compounds that support and feed a healthy gut flora. Vinegar also helps increase populations of healthy gut flora in studies.

We also know that your gut flora has an effect on your weight. Healthy, lean subjects have been shown to have healthy gut flora, while unhealthy subjects have more pathogenic bacteria species.

A study that was published in the *Journal of Nutritional Biochemistry* demonstrated that the combination of vinegar, green tea, and fruit lead to weight loss in obese patients. The polyphenol content in these foods is thought to have a transformative effect on gut microbiota. All of these things are included in this plan to support efficient weight loss.

IMPROVED DIGESTION

Apple cider vinegar improves digestion and is particularly beneficial for people with stomach issues like reflux, bloating, and indigestion. The vinegar improves the pH balance in the stomach, which helps to support the effect of the hydrochloric acid that is released from the stomach cells. This then increases the production and stimulation of the gastric acid secretions, which play an important role in protein, carbohydrate, and fat digestion. This digestive support improves the assimilation of the macro- and micronutrients in meals that are consumed with ACV.

Poor digestion has the consequence of inhibiting the assimilation of nutrients and interfering with the health of the bowel, which can have a strong influence on your well-being and health.

Digestive problems can include bloating, indigestion, flatulence, reflux, constipation, and diarrhea.

BLOATING & INDIGESTION

Bloating and indigestion can be caused by inefficient digestion of protein, carbohydrates, and/or fats in the diet, an unhealthy gut flora, upper digestive infections such as Small Intestinal Bacterial Overgrowth (SIBO), and/or food intolerances. ACV helps to improve these symptoms.

FLATULENCE

Flatulence is often caused by inefficient digestion and poor gut health. Many foods that are more difficult to digest, particularly highly processed foods, are more likely to cause an increase in flatulence.

By improving your diet and consuming apple cider vinegar regularly, you will be able to support a healthier digestive system and reduce flatulence.

Other beneficial foods and drinks for improved digestion include probiotic foods, such as kefir, sauerkraut, or kombucha. You could also take a comprehensive broad-spectrum probiotic.

REFLUX

It may seem strange to recommend ACV as a treatment for acid reflux, particularly when high stomach acid is a contributing factor to acid reflux. As stomach acid makes its way up the esophagus (this is the tube that carries food into your stomach), it causes pain and discomfort. The esophageal tissues are not designed to withstand the higher acid levels that the stomach cells are. Reflux can occur for many reasons, such as poor digestion and stomach health, poor liver health, stomach infections, lack of muscle tone in the lower esophagus, and an abnormally functioning lower esophageal sphincter (LES).

Normal allopathic treatment includes acid neutralizers, proton pump inhibitors, and H2-antagonists. These can reduce the pain and discomfort, but they might also cause other side-effects, such as an increase in respiratory infections, kidney disease, increased hip fractures, and digestive problems like increased bloating, allergies, irregular bowel movements, and digestive discomfort.

Apple cider vinegar can be helpful in cases of reflux and heartburn, since it improves food digestion in the stomach. This improves the passage of food through the stomach and into the intestine for people that may have sluggish digestion. This reduces the time food sits in the stomach and the possibility of regurgitation.

Another contributing factor to reflux is insufficient stomach acid, which may stop the esophageal sphincter from closing adequately, thus allowing food to regurgitate back into the esophagus. It is believed that the LES is a pH-sensitive valve. An increase in acid in the stomach sends a message to the cells to close the sphincter properly, thus reducing the occurrences of reflux. As people age, their stomach acid levels naturally decline, so by consuming ACV, you may increase the acid levels, thus improving digestion and reflux.

Note: ACV can be irritating for some and may irritate your reflux further. It is best to start slowly and observe if there is any aggravation of your symptoms. Start with 1 teaspoon of ACV per glass of water before each meal.

Frequent or constant heartburn, however, can be a serious problem and is the most common symptom of gastroesophageal reflux disease (GERD). It is best to seek medical advice if this is an ongoing condition.

Other helpful tips to reduce reflux—Losing weight can have a dramatic effect on reflux symptoms. Eating smaller, more frequent, healthy meals and avoiding common irritants, such as coffee, nicotine, spicy foods, and fatty meals, can also help.

CONSTIPATION

ACV contains acetic acid, which supports microbial gut health, thus improving stool formation. The malic acid content may also be supportive for constipation. To improve constipation symptoms, mix 2 tablespoons of ACV in warm water 2–3 times daily before meals. You can add lemon and honey if desired to improve the taste.

Other helpful remedies for constipation: You can decrease the frequency of constipation by increasing your fluid intake, exercising frequently, and eating more fruits, vegetables, nuts, seeds and whole grains.

DIARRHEA

In some cases of diarrhea, the intestinal lining may be soothed by small doses of ACV. Consuming ACV regularly may help reduce the likelihood of diarrhea.

ULCERS

This can be tricky, but mixed with an active raw honey (about 1 tablespoon), ACV can offer healing and soothing properties. It may also help to assist with the healing of ulcers.

CANDIDA INFECTIONS

The effects of Candida can be bad breath, lack of energy, UTIs, and digestive issues, along with other possible health issues. ACV contains probiotics and a type of acid that promotes the growth of beneficial bacteria in the digestive system, which help kill off Candida. Remove sugar from your diet and consume 1 tablespoon of apple cider vinegar 3x daily as part of a Candida cleanse.

MORNING SICKNESS

Whether it's in the morning or all day long, pregnancy-related nausea and vomiting can be debilitating. I discovered this trick while pregnant with my second child. Combine 1–3 teaspoons ACV in warm water with a little honey and—BAM—the nausea will subside dramatically. Remember to start slowly with 1 teaspoon and honey, then work your way up with the ACV.

HICCUPS

Apple cider vinegar is a traditional remedy for hiccups, which can be caused by eating too quickly, or from low amounts of stomach acid. Apple cider vinegar can help to restore the acid balance of the stomach and ease this irritating spasm of the diaphragm. To treat hiccups, combine 1 teaspoon of apple cider vinegar and a glass of warm water, and sip it slowly.

INFLAMMATION

Studies show that vinegar has a significant effect on reducing inflammatory conditions by improving the gut flora. The vinegar supports an over-reactive immune system and has been shown to have a significant beneficial effect on asthma and possibly other immune disorders and allergies.

Apple cider vinegar is a good source of polyphenols, which have been shown to help prevent many inflammation-based chronic diseases, such as cardiovascular diseases, cancers, and neurodegenerative diseases like Alzheimer's, osteoporosis, and diabetes.

ALLERGIES

ACV helps to reduce mucus production and allergic reactions by reducing an over-reactive immune system.

SINUS INFECTIONS

Drinking ACV in water can reduce the infection associated with sinus congestion and allergies. The acetic acid helps to thin the mucus.

ANTI-AGING

If you want to help yourself to stay young, then start drinking ACV. Bioactive substances like polyphenols and vitamins in different types of vinegar defend against oxidative stress and can scavenge free radicals, resulting in a potent antioxidant activity. The effect reduces the aging of cells and their degeneration.

URINARY TRACT INFECTIONS

Earl Mindell, M.D., health expert and author of *Dr. Earl Mindell's Amazing Apple Cider Vinegar*, claims ACV can prevent urinary tract infections. Mindell asserts that drinking apple cider vinegar creates a slightly more acidic environment in the urinary tract and creates slightly more acidic urine, both of which help to discourage pathogenic bacterial growth. This may only work as an infection prevention (not a cure) for people who are predisposed to repeated urinary infections. If you believe you have an infection, you should see your doctor.

Using Apple Cider Vinegar Topically

SORE THROAT

If you can feel a sore throat coming on, gargling ACV can stop it in its tracks. Try gargling ¼ cup of ACV with ¼ cup of water every hour. This acts as a topical antiseptic and anti-inflammatory.

BRUISES

Apple cider vinegar has anti-inflammatory properties; using an apple cider vinegar compress on a bruise can help fade the discoloration.

BAD BREATH

Due to its antiseptic properties, apple cider vinegar makes a wonderful remedy for bad breath, also known as halitosis. Simply add 1 tablespoon of ACV to a cup of water, and gargle the mixture in your mouth for 10 seconds at a time. Repeat until the cup is empty.

FOOT ODOR

Fill a small foot bath with warm water and add ⅓ cup of ACV, and then let your feet soak in this mixture for 15 minutes once per week.

TOENAIL FUNGAL INFECTIONS

Antibacterial and antifungal compounds in apple cider vinegar make it a great natural cure for skin and toenail fungus. Simply rub some ACV on the fungus 2xs daily or do a regular foot bath as instructed above.

AGE OR SUN SPOTS

Apple cider vinegar contains sulfur that fights the effects of aging, which makes it suitable for treating age spots. Be patient. This process can take some time, but with repeated use it can really reduce them.

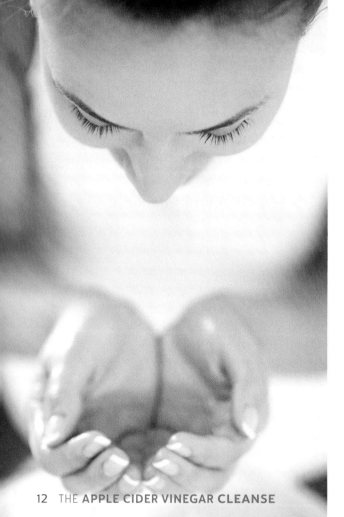

SUNBURN

Mother of vinegar has been demonstrated to have a therapeutic effect on burns due to its antibacterial and soothing properties. Add 1 cup of ACV to a full bathtub and soak for 20 minutes to help relieve sunburn. You can add some anti-inflammatory essential oils, such as lavender and chamomile, to further soothe the inflamed skin.

SKIN PROBLEMS

Apple cider vinegar is a great natural skin toner that can reduce skin blemishes and acne; it also supports a healthy skin pH. Apple cider vinegar is a great astringent and acts as a natural antiseptic, which helps to reduce skin infections and inflammation of the skin.

Mix 1 part ACV to 2 parts water and dab it on your face and pimples with cotton balls. If you have sensitive skin, it may be advisable to dilute this mixture down further to 1 part vinegar to 3–4 parts water. Using a test area is the best option initially.

ITCHY SKIN

Itchy skin can be cause by allergies, stress, infections, dry skin, and poor liver heath. ACV may help reduce this itch; just add ¼ cup of ACV to 1 cup of water and apply it to the skin via a spray bottle or a cloth. I remember having a case of hives and jumping in an ACV bath to help relieve the skin irritation—it relieved the itch quickly.

FACIAL MASK

Mix 1 tablespoon of apple cider vinegar and bentonite clay; add 1 tablespoon of raw honey. Apply to skin. Leave this detoxifying, deep-pore treatment on for 10–15 minutes before rinsing off with warm water. This will make 2–3 masks that you can store in the fridge.

STINGS

Apple cider vinegar can soothe a wasp sting. The vinegar's acid converts certain toxins in the venom to less toxic compounds. Dousing your skin with vinegar is also an effective folk remedy for most jellyfish stings, as it deactivates venom cells. It's important to apply cider vinegar to a wasp or jellyfish sting with a cotton ball or soft pad.

WARTS

Put apple cider vinegar topically on a wart, and then cover it with a bandage; leave the bandage on overnight. You may see results in 1–2 weeks, or it could take a little longer.

VARICOSE VEINS

ACV is great for easing the swelling of the veins, so they are less noticeable and less painful. Combine equal parts ACV and a natural body moisturizer. Apply morning and night, rubbing it in well. Improvement can be seen in about 1 month depending on the severity.

SNORING

There is some belief that ACV may help reduce snoring when consumed regularly.

NATURAL DEODORANT

ACV can help to adjust the skin's pH level, which helps to eliminate odor-causing bacteria. For body odor, simply wipe underarms once each morning with undiluted apple cider vinegar using a cotton ball, tissue, or spritzer. Remember: it is advisable to test an area of your skin initially and for sensitive skin to dilute the ACV with water.

HEALTHY SHINY HAIR

Beauty blogs suggest that adding one part vinegar to one part water and using it as you would conditioner—that is, applying it to your hair and letting it soak in for between 5–15 minutes before rinsing can help improve the health of your hair.

It is also said to reduce dandruff because it helps to balance the pH of the scalp and reduces any infection that may be present on the scalp that can contribute to dandruff. Mix equal parts of vinegar to water and leave it on the scalp for 10–15 minutes; then rinse off. Repeat this process twice weekly. Alternatively, you can add this to a spritzer bottle and spray it on the hair and scalp. Leave on for 15 minutes to an hour, and then rinse it out.

TEETH WHITENING

Apple cider vinegar is a cheap and simple way to restore your teeth's natural white sheen. Apple cider vinegar helps remove stains and kills bacteria in your mouth and gums. All you need to do is gargle with apple cider vinegar every morning, rinse with water, and then brush your teeth as usual.

Apple Cider Vinegar Household Uses

NATURAL FOOD PRESERVATIVE

ACV can help prevent foods from spoiling quickly, and it can also reduce oxidation of fresh food. Sprinkling ACV over your avocado, apple, or fresh food will prevent it from going brown and will reduce the likelihood of it becoming contaminated with E. coli and other pathogens.

FRUIT AND VEGETABLE WASH

Soaking fruits and vegetables in 1 part vinegar and 3 parts water can reduce and kill any possible pathogens found on fresh fruits and vegetables. It can also extend the life of the produce

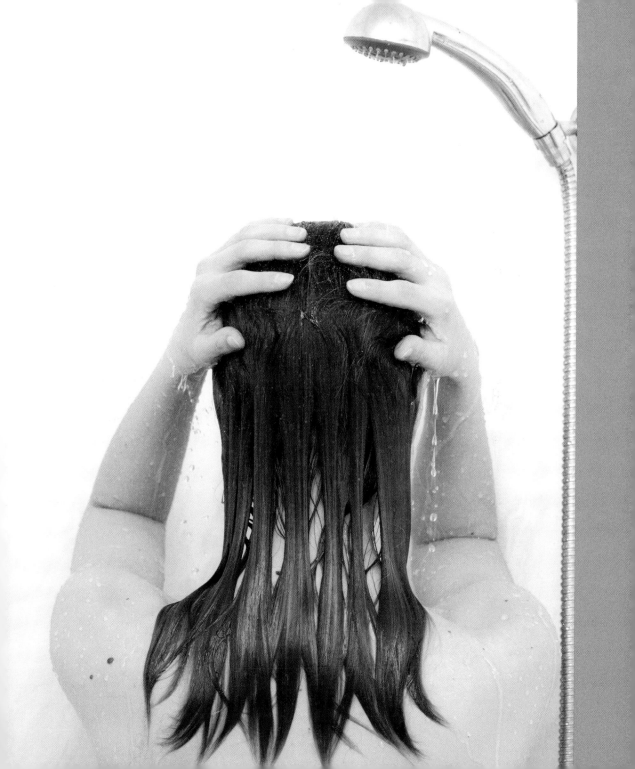

by killing any fungal and yeast infestations that may be present on the surface. This can also be useful for anyone that may be immune compromised to ensure clean, fresh produce.

Another fun tip is to add a spoonful of cider vinegar to boiling vegetables, as this helps them retain their color.

UNCLOGGING DRAINS

Commercial drain cleaners are dangerous and can have environmental and health consequences, such as respiratory damage and other health concerns. To clear a drain the all-natural way, make a solution by sprinkling ½ cup of baking soda into your drain, and then follow it with 1 cup of ACV. Allow it to foam, and then flush the drain with hot water. After 5 minutes, flush it again with cold water. This solution is not only better for your health, but it's also better for the environment.

WOOD POLISH

Another known use for ACV is in the conditioning of wood. A concoction of half a cup of any vegetable oil with half a cup of apple cider vinegar is said to create a polish that will clean and treat any wooden furniture or surfaces and remove water stains.

SURFACE ANTISEPTIC

ACV can be used to clean household surfaces and to act as a natural, nontoxic, environmentally friendly household cleaner. A study at the University of North Carolina has shown that vinegar helps to kill surface germs, such as E. coli and S. aureus.

Fill a spray bottle with 50% water and 50% ACV, and then spray surfaces and counters to clean them.

PET CARE

ACV can help to fight fleas on dogs. Create a bath of half water and half ACV, and soak your pet in a tub. Do this once a day for several weeks to rid your pet of a flea infestation. This can also be given to them in their water to assist with digestion, healthy gut flora, and the reduction of any inflammatory conditions.

WEED KILLER

Clear out problematic weeds with a vinegar-based herbicide spray. Combine the undiluted vinegar, orange oil, and liquid soap. Using a spray bottle, shake well and spot-spray the herbicide where weeds grow. This recipe calls for ACV, but for an even stronger spray, "Dirt Doctor" Howard Garrett recommends using white vinegar with 10% acidity.

- 1 gallon of ACV
- 1 ounce orange oil or d-limonene
- 1 teaspoon liquid soap

WASHING CLOTHES

Vinegar can be a good stain remover. White vinegar and ACV both work well. Soak clothes in vinegar or pour it in the wash to help remove stains, lint, and grime.

DETOX AND RELAX BATH SOAK

Add 2 cups of ACV to a hot bathtub. Add 1 cup of Epsom salts, 5 drops of lavender, and 3 drops of geranium or chamomile (optional). Soak for 20–30 minutes and leave the solution sitting on the skin for at least 10–12 hours.

chapter 2. What Is the **ACV Cleanse?**

In the cleanse program, I have included the regular consumption of apple cider vinegar. The Cleanse consists of a healthy eating and juicing plan to help reset your health and lose any excess pounds.

The addition of the ACV gives you the upper hand in improving your health and losing weight in the most effective way possible.

There is exciting new research that supports the use of apple cider in weight loss programs. The studies have found that drinking this specific type of vinegar causes a considerable decrease in overall body weight, waistline circumference, and triglyceride levels. Some of these studies have been done over a 12-week trial. Once the Cleanse finishes, it is advised that you continue consuming ACV regularly to support your overall health and continued success.

With the addition of the ACV to the Cleanse, you will be able to assist your blood sugar levels, reduce the over production of insulin, and improve satiety. In a study of the effects of ACV on appetite regulation, it was found that participants felt fuller and more satisfied when consuming bread and vinegar together than when eating bread alone. The Cleanse allows you to reap these same benefits by consuming regular doses of ACV with a diet of juices, smoothies, and fruit-and-vegetable-based meals.

What Are the Benefits of a Cleanse?

This is a frequent and very important question! A cleanse is a period of time when you are actively increasing your nutrition and reducing your exposure to unhealthy foods, beverages, and environmental factors. It's a special time for healing when you can work toward rejuvenating your health, reducing cravings, and shedding excess body weight.

Cleanse periods are great ways to jump-start a permanent, healthy eating pattern. The cleanse process supports your focus on nutritionally dense meals and excludes foods that are not so nutritious so that you can enjoy a period of complete avoidance of unhealthy foods.

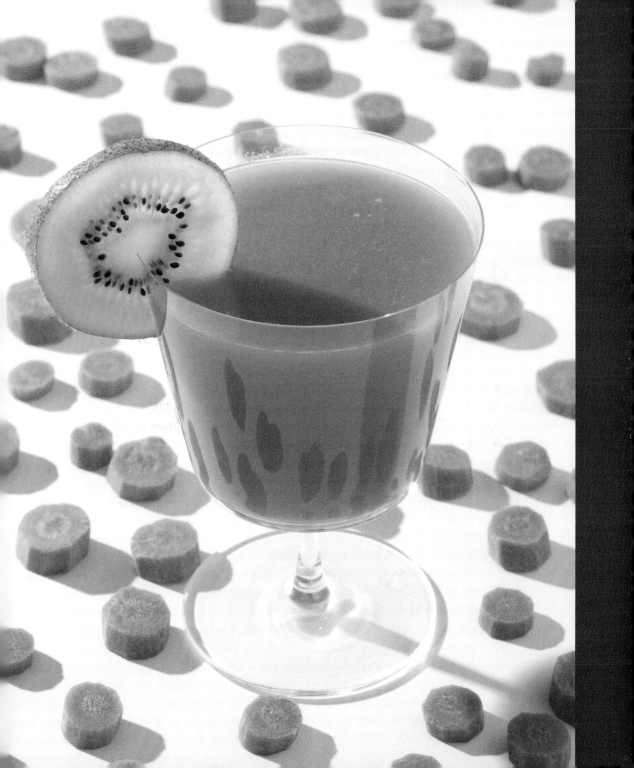

While completing a mostly liquid cleanse, your digestive system will be working at a reduced level, so the body can enjoy easily assimilated nutrients and focus its energy on cell renewal and other health changes. When you complete a cleanse, some of the first positive symptoms experienced will be improved skin appearance and improved energy levels as the nutrients will be replenished in the body and the skin. The skin is the last place that nutrients tend to be delivered, so when we saturate our bodies with intense levels of antioxidants and plant compounds, it starts to show up in our skin and our eyes very quickly. This is often what people will comment on the most once they have started their ACV Cleanse.

The initial stages of the ACV Cleanse may be difficult, but within a few days or less your cravings will reduce and you will be feeling lighter and more energized. These changes will also support healthier food choices after the cleanse period has finished, thus giving you continued benefits and improved health.

Cleanse programs also help to reduce your overall intake of unhealthy foods, since your cravings will be reduced and your satiety signals will be more effective to help you stop eating when you're full.

Why Cleanse?

Some people claim that you do not need to cleanse the body because your body is cleansing itself all of the time. This is true! Detoxification is one of the body's most basic and normal functions. Your liver, kidneys, bowels, lymphatic system, and skin are constantly detoxifying your body and eliminating chemicals and waste via your sweat, urine, and feces. For these detox processes to work optimally, you need to reduce health burdens where possible and improve your level of nutrition.

There are certain plant compounds, vitamins, and minerals that are vital for these detoxification processes to work optimally. If you are lacking in any of these specialized nutrients, you will not be able to efficiently support detoxification. This can lead to fatigue, poor health, and weight struggles.

If we burden our health with exposure to too many toxins and too few nutrients, then we will inevitably suffer the consequences.

The Centers for Disease Control and Prevention conducted the Fourth National Report on Human Exposure to Environmental Chemicals. On average, the CDC's report found 212 chemicals in people's blood or urine, 75 of which had never before been measured in the U.S. population. It is known that many of the detected chemicals can be harmful to human health and capable of contributing to chronic disease and other health concerns. Considering these facts, it's hard to escape the probability that our bodies are under enormous strain. Supporting yourself with periods of cleansing will give you significantly improved health outcomes.

We are unfortunately exposed to many environmental contaminates, such as:

- Herbicides
- Pesticides
- Insecticides
- Petrochemicals
- Hair dyes & beauty products that may contain carcinogenic chemicals
- Cleaning products
- Medications, particularly painkillers and other narcotics
- Air pollutants
- Synthetic fragrances
- Plastic substances, such as BPA and phthalates

Combined with poor diets, which may include:

- Processed oils
- Artificial sweeteners
- Food additives
- Preservatives
- Excess refined carbohydrates
- Excess sugar
- Trans-fats
- Excess alcohol

All of these factors contribute to poor health, liver disease, fatigue, immune diseases, chronic inflammation, and weight gain.

It's important to let your body have a breather every once in a while to allow healing, a reduction in inflammation, and a regeneration of healthy tissues to occur. While it is NOT possible to completely eliminate toxin exposure from all sources, there are ways to minimize exposure.

We know that the liver, the digestive system, and other organ systems can often regenerate from a state of disease to healthy functioning tissue. For example, a lack of fresh vegetables and too many processed foods can cause a fatty liver; this can be reversed with improved nutrition and a healthy lifestyle. A cleanse is also a great opportunity to help retrain your body and increase your desires for healthy foods and reduce unhealthy food cravings.

What Happens During Detoxification?

Detoxification is the metabolic process of removing unwanted compounds from the body. These unwanted compounds can be foreign environmental toxins (xenobiotics), or they can be a by-product of normal metabolism, such as hormones, inflammatory molecules, and old cells. The liver is the primary detoxification organ, along with the intestines, kidneys, skin, and bowel.

Detoxification includes neutralizing and eliminating waste from the digestion of food, cellular respiration, and immune complexes, along with the elimination of environmental pollutants.

The process of detoxification removes toxins by converting fat-soluble toxic compounds into water-soluble compounds that can be eliminated easily. The liver also synthesizes and removes bile that is full of fat-soluble toxins and cholesterol and eliminates unwanted chemicals via an enzymatic process that includes three phases.

These three phases involve a series of enzymatic reactions that neutralize and solubilize toxins and transport them to secretory organs (such as the bowels, skin, and kidneys) so that they can be excreted from the body. Liver health and proper detoxification are central to the body's homeostatic balance.

In Phase 1 of liver detoxification, enzymes that require specific nutrients begin converting these lipid soluble compounds into unstable intermediate compounds that are more reactive and more toxic. They are metabolized by the 2nd phase of liver detoxification, where they become completely water soluble and suitable for transportation out of the body.

If the Phase 1 detoxification of the liver is metabolizing at a faster rate than Phase 2, which is often the case in sluggish liver function, then these partially converted metabolites that build up can cause increased free radical damage, posing a health concern due to increased inflammation and accelerated aging.

Factors that can increase Phase 1 and decrease Phase 2 of detoxification are a poor diet, age, alcohol, medications, drugs, smoking, disease, and genetic polymorphisms. Good nutrition and a healthy diet provide the backbone for these normal phases to function effectively and efficiently.

Research literature written by Dr. DeAnn Liska, Ph.D. and published in the *Alternative Medicine Review* suggests an association between impaired detoxification and disease. This is especially the case with increased Phase 1 and/or decreased Phase 2, which are associated with an increase in diseases such as cancer, Parkinson's disease, lupus, fibromyalgia, chronic fatigue, and other immune dysfunction syndromes.

In Phase 2 detoxification, six processes occur. These processes are acylation, glucuronidation, glutathione conjugation, methylation, sulfation, and acetylation. Each of these pathways requires specific nutrients to function efficiently.

As you can see, with an inadequate intake of nutrients, a lack of healthy fresh food, and too much inflammation, there will certainly be impairment in function. A cleanse allows these pathways to function properly, allowing for good health.

Perhaps these last few paragraphs may have contained more information than you wanted or needed to know, but believe it or not, I have a point. The metabolism of the liver is very complicated, and it requires a diverse array of nutrients and plant compounds, combined with as little negative environmental factors as possible, to work optimally rather than sluggishly. A cleanse absolutely gives it a service that it needs, with the added bonus of your learning how to eat and drink to support good health in the long term.

More on Liver Health

There is a reason why I have such respect and adoration for this hard-working organ; it is involved in more than 200 chemical processes in the body and is often nicknamed the "General of the Army." The liver filters approximately 50 oz. (1.5 L) of blood every minute and plays a role in nearly every bodily function.

The liver is responsible for energy production, nutrient storage, eliminating waste, producing bile for fat digestion, controlling cholesterol levels, monitoring natural hormonal balances, producing immune factors to fight infections, and detoxifying the blood by filtering out toxins as discussed.

A very common health issue that effects many people is fatty liver disease, a condition in which the liver contains an excessive amount of fat and the healthy liver cells are partly replaced with areas of unhealthy fats. The liver cells and the spaces in the liver are filled with fat, so the liver becomes slightly enlarged and can have a yellow, greasy appearance.

Causes of a fatty liver include excess alcohol, diabetes, poor blood sugar control or insulin resistance, taking many medications for long periods of time (polypharmacy), poor nutrition, eating too many processed foods, obesity or carrying excess weight around your torso, or simply being an apple shaped person.

Symptoms associated with poor liver function include:

- Pain or discomfort under the right ribcage
- Indigestion
- Bloating
- Intolerance to fatty foods
- Fatigue
- Chronic skin itching
- Poor concentration
- Intolerance to heat
- Gallstones
- Elevated LDL cholesterol
- Fat around the upper abdomen (indicates visceral fat)
- Weight gain
- Sugar imbalances
- Food cravings
- Increased chemical sensitivities and allergies
- Dark circles around the eyes

I believe that comments claiming we do not need to cleanse are purely based on an inadequate understanding on the complexities of how the liver functions and what optimizes its function versus what sabotages its function. If you are very healthy, and you always lived an exceptionally healthy lifestyle, then perhaps you don't need to cleanse. But I think everyone can benefit from a period of restriction and improved plant nutrition with the essential inclusion of ACV and other super nutrient-dense food.

A wide variety of dietary components have been shown to activate and increase the activity of Phase 2 liver detoxification, such as:

- Epigallocatechin gallate (EGCG) in green tea
- Curcumin, a compound found in turmeric, increases liver detoxification, supports gallbladder emptying, and protects the liver against alcohol damage.
- Betaine, a compound found in beets (beetroot) supports methylation Phase 2 detox pathways.
- Dietary organosulfur and indole-3-carbinol containing vegetables, such as garlic, onions, cabbage, kale, radishes, Brussels sprouts, broccoli, and cauliflower, support and stimulate sulfation and glutathione conjugation.
- Vitamin C enhances glutathione conjugation and acetylation.
- Vitamin B is required for many Phase 2 functions.
- Magnesium, found in dark leafy greens, is essential for methylation.
- Free amino acids like methionine, glycine, cysteine, and taurine

When the body is in a state of inflammation, our detoxification pathways become impaired. To support the natural pathways of detoxification, we also need to provide the antioxidants and plant compounds that not only improve detoxification but also reduce systemic and tissue inflammation to allow for detoxification to occur.

How many people suffer from inflammatory health conditions? These conditions contribute to impaired liver detoxification pathways. People suffering from chronic arthritis, diabetes, heart disease, immune conditions, and obesity will have impaired detoxification, thus further contributing to chronic disease and inflammation; it becomes a destructive cascading situation.

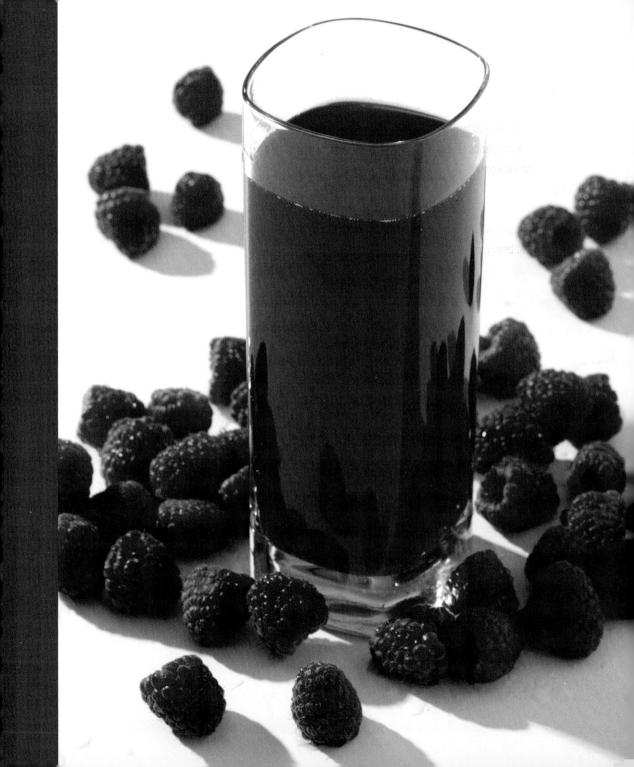

Antioxidants found in fruits and vegetables contain a myriad of plant compounds that have very strong anti-inflammatory effects. Ginger, turmeric, pineapple, berries, cherries, citrus, carrots, watermelon, red cabbage, sweet potato, and more all contain specialized compounds that provide anti-inflammatory effects which can help to reduce and possibly reverse diseases.

Research finds that certain foods and nutrients are associated with the regulation of detoxification enzymes, leading to more enzymes being present and faster rates of xenobiotic detoxification.

This allows the natural biochemical detoxification pathways to work more efficiently with a reduced workload. When you provide the body and the liver with proper nutrition, all the natural biochemical detoxifications pathways are supported.

Calorie Restriction and the Associated Health Benefits

Dietary restriction and fasting have been around for thousands of years, particularly for religious, health, healing, and cultural reasons. Traditional cultures all around the world have used fasting and nutritional cleansing as an integral part preventative health care plans. It is also used for inflammatory disease states and poor health; studies indicate that periods of fasting and calorie restriction have been shown to support healthier and longer lives with less disease and reduced cellular aging. Yes, that means you can look younger for longer! Cultures that fast intermittently throughout their lives have been shown to have healthier, longer lives than people who never break from continuous eating.

Fasting and calorie restriction are recommended to allow the body to heal. The traditional ideology is that since very little energy is required to digest food, this energy can be better utilized by the body for regeneration and healing.

Eating constantly is not something that serves us well. Today, more Americans are obese than just overweight. Something clearly isn't working.

There is scientific research to support the long-term health benefits of intermittent fasting and calorie restriction. Mark P. Mattson, chief of the laboratory of neurosciences at the National Institute on Aging, says, "In normal healthy subjects, moderate fasting such as cutting back on calories a couple of days a week will have health benefits for almost anybody." Mattson is among the leading researchers on the effects of calorie restriction on the brain.

Dr. Valter Longo, Professor of Gerontology and the Biological Sciences at the University of California, says fasting "flips a regenerative switch in our immune systems," which prompts stem cells to create brand new white blood cells, essentially regenerating the entire immune system. This can be particularly helpful for people who are undergoing chemotherapy and who have cancer and other immune diseases. Studies show that calorie restriction has a profound impact on age-related diseases including a reduced risk of cancer, neurodegenerative disorders, autoimmune diseases, cardiovascular disease, and type 2 diabetes.

Animal studies suggest calorie restriction may reduce the risk of cancer by slowing the growth of abnormal cells, may reduce cognitive decline in diseases like Alzheimer's disease and Parkinson's disease, and may even increase life expectancy.

Intermittent fasting appears to offer the same advantages as long-term calorie restriction, which is defined as eating at regular times but consuming 25% to 30% fewer calories than what is recommended for that person based on their age, size, and gender. This can be easily achieved by filling up on nutrient-dense, low-calorie foods such as vegetables and some fruits. The ACV 7-Day Cleanse provides this calorie restriction, while also supporting appetite control and satiety.

Based on these results, following the ACV Cleanse will offer an array of health benefits in the longterm.

Health Benefits of the 7-Day ACV Cleanse

The ACV Cleanse helps you take the next step forward to reset your internal systems and encourages your food intake to be 100% plant based and healthy to support improved detoxification, blood sugar balance, weight loss, and improved energy and mood.

In the many years I have worked with detox programs and juice fasts, I have seen so many dramatic changes. I have worked with thousands of people to help them achieve the health results that they deserve by following these guidelines.

In my experience, I've seen a long list of health improvements from making these changes. The improvements include:

- Reduced muscle aches and pains
- Reduce arthritis pain with improved mobility

- Improved digestion
- Improved sleep
- Reduced headaches and migraines
- Increased energy levels
- Stronger immune systems to fight those pesky colds and flus
- Improved skin complexion and reversal of many skin conditions
- Improved liver health
- Weight loss
- Improved blood pressure readings
- Improved cholesterol levels
- Blood sugar improvements in cases of diabetes, insulin resistance, and hypoglycemia
- Improved immune functions in autoimmune diseases and post-viral syndrome
- Improved mood, cognition, and mental clarity
- Increased motivation and will power
- Improved gut health and an increase in healthy, beneficial bugs
- A permanent kick-off into a healthy lifestyle

It sounds pretty amazing, doesn't it? Well it is, and it never ceases to amaze me when I see such great results!

Preparing for Your ACV 7-Day Cleanse

It is very important that you prepare yourself for your 7-Day ACV Cleanse! To prepare, it is suggested that you avoid consuming any unhealthy foods and limiting other recommended foods listed below. This is just as important as doing the 7-Day Cleanse to allow your body to adjust to new foods, flavors, portions sizes, macronutrient balance, and caloric reductions. It will help you get the best results possible.

It can be tempting to simply follow your normal eating patterns and then dive straight into the ACV Cleanse on Day 1. I have even heard of some people having that last hurrah meal before starting a cleanse; unfortunately, this just makes it more difficult to begin and harder to stick to. If we eat poorly before the cleanse, our cravings will be elevated and we will feel more hungry. We are also more likely to experience the negative side effects of reducing your calories, fats, sugars, and caffeine.

Diving into 7-Day ACV Cleanse without any preparation just gives you less of a chance to be successful. If the plan becomes a struggle, then people are more likely to give up. Alternatively, if you prepare yourself adequately and set yourself up for success, then you will enjoy the process and experience greater results. You will be more likely to achieve your health goals and be on your way to a healthier lifestyle.

Getting prepared can be the **single most productive step** you can take to make this as enjoyable as it should be and to give you your best results!

Foods and beverages to eliminate during the pre-Cleanse, the ACV Cleanse, and post-Cleanse period include:

- Alcohol
- Coffee and regular black tea
- Sugar and all other sweeteners (except for a little honey and Stevia)
- Soft drinks
- Food additives, artificial flavors, and preservatives

Follow these suggestions 7 days leading up to your Cleanse (pre-Cleanse)

- **Avoid alcohol, sugar, coffee, processed packaged foods, fast food, deep-fried foods, food additives, and preservatives.**
- Avoiding packaged foods is a great starting point for healthier eating. Shopping largely around the perimeter of the grocery store (or better yet, shopping at your local farmers market), is an excellent step forward.
- Reducing the portion size of your meals is also important before the 7-Day Cleanse to help make the transition into the plan easier. This is a great time to also start practicing mindful eating and start paying attention to the way food makes you feel.

- After you ate (or while you ate) in the past, consider how you felt physically, emotionally, and mentally. After your meal or snack did you experience gas, acid reflux, or bloating? When you ate sugar or refined carbohydrates (such as white bread, crackers, or pasta) did you notice that you crashed 30 minutes later, feeling irritable? These are important things to be aware of.

Suggestions during your 7 day pre-Cleanse period:

Days 1–3

AVOID

- Sugar
- Processed and packaged foods
- Food additives
- All vegetable oil blends, hydrogenated oils, and vegetable fats

Read the ingredients of any foods that you are considering eating and become familiar with brands and food labels. Long ingredient lists are often warning signs that it's not a good choice.

Processed foods include anything with an ingredient list that requires chemistry knowledge, or a list that contains numbers or any words that indicate the product is not from nature.

CONSUME Instead . . .

- Healthy organic grass-fed meats, poultry, eggs, nuts, seeds, legumes, whole grains, fruits, and vegetable-based meals and snacks.

Days 4–5

AVOID

- Red meat
- All dairy products (including butter, cream, milk, yogurt, and kefir)
- Gluten-containing grains, such as wheat, rye, barley, kamut, or spelt.

This is an excellent time to evaluate whether gluten is a problem in your diet. As a practitioner, I have seen so many health problems resolved once gluten has been eliminated from the diet, including in people who have tested negative to all the normal gluten tests that are currently available. See more on this below. You can consume gluten-free grains, such as quinoa, wild rice, teff, buckwheat, or brown rice.

CONSUME instead . . .

- Organic poultry, organic eggs, wild fish, and vegetarian proteins. Vegetarian proteins include legumes that are well prepared if tolerated (see more on this), nuts, seeds, and gluten-free grains as an alternative protein source.
- Coconut oil, cold-pressed olive oil, and avocado oil

Days 6–7

AVOID

- All animal products (including fish, eggs, and poultry)

Remember on these days to start enjoying some of the suggested recipes and start drinking vegetable juices and smoothies daily. In the pre-Cleanse period, you want your diet to be filled with an abundance of color and variety.

CONSUME Instead . . .

- Fruits and vegetables as suggested
- Nuts, seeds, and healthy gluten-free whole grains and legumes

A good guide to follow daily is to consume at least:

- 2 vegetable-based dishes daily pre-Cleanse—juices, smoothies, soups, salad and other vegetable-based dishes
- 2 servings of fruit—a serving of fruit is approximately 1 cup

The recipe section contains some great recipes you can make!

Guidelines for the 7-Day ACV Cleanse

On this cleanse you will be consuming only fruits and vegetables in the form of juices, smoothies, salads, soups, and other vegetable- and fruit-based meals. Some healthy oils, herbs, and spices will also be included.

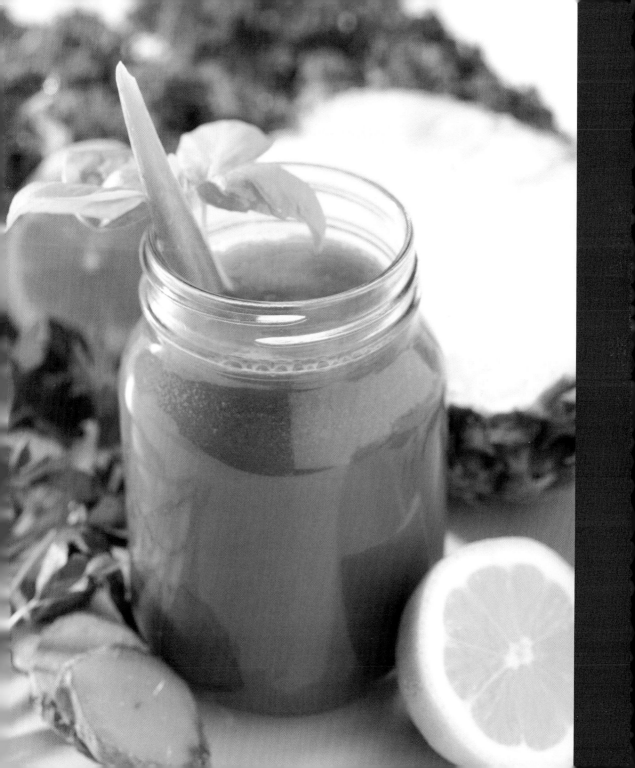

Foods to ELIMINATE completely in the 7-Day ACV Cleanse period:

- Grains (including all breads, crackers, crisp breads, cereals, pasta, baked goods)
- Nuts
- Seeds (except hemp seeds and chia seeds)
- Legumes
- Animal products, including meat, eggs, fish, and seafood
- All dairy products, including goat and sheep dairy, milk, cream, cheese, yogurt, and kefir

What foods are INCLUDED on the ACV 7-Day Cleanse:

- Fruits
- Vegetables
- Herbs
- Spices
- Extra-virgin olive oil, avocado oil, coconut oil
- Chia and hemp seeds
- ACV

Optional Superfood additions:

- Spirulina, coconut water kefir, kombucha, and psyllium husks.

CAFFEINE DURING THE CLEANSE

Although there are studies that suggest that coffee offers a range of health benefits, it can be beneficial to have a break from your regular black tea or coffee for a short period of time. You can resume drinking it once the post-cleanse period is finished if you so choose. After the 7-Day Cleanse, your taste buds and palate can change, and you may prefer herbal teas or a warm lemon and apple cider vinegar drink as your new preferred start of the day beverage.

I suggest purchasing a certified organic coffee whenever possible, preferably from within the country where you live, to ensure that it is not fumigated with methyl bromide; approximately 90% of the coffee in the U.S. is treated with methyl bromide for up to 8 hours.

Coffee, unfortunately, is also sprayed heavily with pesticides and is often grown in countries that have relaxed laws with little control over pesticides and environmental contaminants. To reduce your body's chemical intake, it is best to purchase and drink certified organic coffee.

It is advisable to only drink 1–2 cups of coffee per day to maintain good health post-Cleanse. Coffee can easily deliver too much caffeine and can cause short-term effects like muscle twitching, increased heart rate, reduced blood flow to the stomach, more sugar released into the bloodstream, anxiety, sleep disorders, and restlessness. The amount of caffeine needed to cause these reactions is dependent on many factors, such as tolerance, age, weight, sex, and liver health.

Many people think that caffeine doesn't affect their sleep, but it certainly can contribute to shorter sleep cycles and restless sleep, less time spent dreaming, and feeling restless and fatigued during the day.

Freshly brewed coffee contains 75–200 mg of caffeine per cup, while instant coffee can contain 27–173 mg. Black tea averages 14–70 mg of caffeine per cup, while green tea averages only 25–45 mg per cup. These levels depend on growing conditions and other factors.

Drinking green tea can be an easier way to support your energy levels while cutting your caffeine consumption down. Reducing caffeine suddenly can cause withdrawal symptoms such as headaches, migraines, lethargy, poor energy, and a poor mood.

TIPS FOR WEANING YOURSELF OFF CAFFEINE PRE-CLEANSE

In the days leading up to the 7-Day ACV Cleanse, you can slowly start reducing your caffeine intake down by a quarter or half each day and substitute an herbal tea, juice, green tea, or water.

If you normally consume 4 cups of coffee or black tea per day, then reduce this to 3 cups. The following day, consume 2. Continue to drop the number of servings until you get to zero cups. You should ensure that you are drinking plenty of fluids. By reducing your intake of caffeine slowly, you are more likely to avoid any withdrawal symptoms.

If you choose to consume green tea, then try to keep it to 1–2 cups per day, preferably in the early part of the day, and move onto herbal tea for the rest of the day. You can purchase caffeine-free green tea if you would like to enjoy the health benefits associated with green tea without the caffeine.

Moving to green tea or matcha tea can provide extra health benefits, such as weight loss due to an increase in thermogenesis and promotion of fat oxidation, enhanced antioxidant intake, cognitive enhancement, cancer prevention, and a reduction in other inflammatory degeneratory diseases. These benefits can also be found in decaf tea, though to a lesser extent.

Getting adequate rest, combined with staying well-nourished and hydrated, will have the greatest effects on your energy levels during each stage of the cleanse program.

Eating More Mindfully During the Cleanse and Beyond

Eating slowly and chewing your food more thoroughly can reduce over-eating and improve digestion. Studies show that consuming food slowly improves weight loss due to improved satiety. If this does not come naturally to you, then consider these steps:

- Put down your knife and fork between mouthfuls.
- Chew your food until it becomes liquefied.
- Eat without distractions. This means you should eat away from screens like your TV, computers, tablets or phones. Studies show that people eat up to twice as much when distracted.
- Don't eat when you're in a hurry or feeling stressed. This often leaves you with indigestion and frequently leads to eating more than you otherwise would have.
- Avoid eating when feeling emotional, as this perpetuates emotional eating that can lead to poor choices and over-consumption. Find an another activity to support yourself, such as a book, a good chat with a supportive person, a nap, a bath, or anything else that helps you to relax.

Remember that the first few mouthfuls are the most enjoyable, and the more you eat something, the less the enjoyment you will experience from each bite. Savor those first few mouthfuls. Notice the texture, aroma, and flavor. It's important to be present and mindful when eating to ensure maximum health and weight loss. Remember to always be present in the moment without judgment.

Tips for Success on the 7-Day Cleanse

Get prepared
Successful eating patterns involve some shopping, prepping and organizing. This is the area I see people fall short on the most when it comes to long-term success. They get busy; they haven't thought about it, and then before they know it they are starving and ready to eat anything. To increase your success, plan ahead; everything will be easier.

Don't skip meals
Even if you're not particularly hungry, it is important to consume the suggested meals, particularly the juices, to ensure you get the results you want. If you skip the meals or juices, you will be more likely to become hungrier later in the day or even the next day. Cravings will increase along with your appetite. This will make the plan more difficult to follow.

Follow the menu as closely as possible
This ensures a variety of nutrients and a lack of boredom. This is also an excellent opportunity to learn some new healthy kitchen skills.

Stay hydrated
Not drinking enough water is a common mistake. Dehydration will increase your hunger and reduce your metabolism. Even if you don't feel thirsty, you might experience other symptoms like fatigue, lethargy, muscle spasms, cramps, and body aches. For every two glasses of water you drink, your metabolism increases by 30%. This can have a significant impact on your weight-loss goals.

Avoid thinking about deprivation; think about the gains
Thoughts of deprivation can set you up to fail; if you focus on all the foods you "can't have," you'll actually crave those foods or beverages more! It's important to focus on what you CAN have and what you can GAIN. You'll learn more about this in the emotional eating section.

Slip-ups
If you slip up, get back into the plan with the next suggested meal or get straight back to where you left off. Often, people worry that once they have eaten something officially off the menu, they have ruined all their good work. That's not true! By getting back into it, you are supporting yourself now and practicing better eating habits for the future. Just keep going and you will succeed!

How to Incorporate ACV into the Plan and Your Diet

Start by adding 1 teaspoon of ACV to a cup of water and drink it once a day as you're leading up to the ACV Cleanse. Then, increase the amount of vinegar per serving, and drink this mixture more frequently.

Once you get to the beginning of the Cleanse, you should ideally be consuming up to 1–2 tablespoons of vinegar in a cup of water three times a day; this can also be added to your meals. The menu plan lists 1 tablespoon as the suggestion, but if you can tolerate it, then you can move up to 2 tablespoons on rising and with lunch and dinner.

To kick-start your metabolism and increase the feeling of fullness, it's best to drink ACV about 15–30 minutes before your meal or during the meal.

ACV is very acidic, so you need to dilute it to protect your teeth, throat, and the lining of your stomach. **Don't drink undiluted ACV!**

Why Juices for Some Meals?

Juice is one of the most nutrient-dense meals you can consume. As you can imagine, juices allow you to ingest large quantities of fruits and vegetables in an easy to digest form. In most cases it would be impossible to consume that amount of produce in one sitting; juicing makes it possible.

Juices can also be a great way to ingest loads of vegetables that you normally wouldn't eat because you can consume them mixed in with fruits and other vegetables that you prefer to consume. Greens, for example, can be consumed easily with apples, pineapple, and sweet vegetables such as carrots and beets.

Including an extra 5–8 servings of fruit and vegetables in one large glass of juice certainly offers enormous health benefits, as a higher fruit and vegetable intake increases well-being and helps reduce the chances of developing a chronic disease.

Points of Concern for Some People When it Comes to Juicing

Sugar content—It is important to be aware that some juices can be too high in naturally occurring sugars, so it's important to make juices from a mostly vegetable base. You can add some fruits or sweeter vegetables to make it enjoyable. A good guideline is to consume 80% vegetables and 20% fruit over the course of the day. This can be adjusted for each individual and is not an exact science. Some days on the plan vary slightly.

Everyone's sweet palate varies. One juice may not be palatable to one person as it's too strong in greens while this same juice may be too sweet for the next person. It's a good idea to always adjust a recipe to your preference to make sure you'll stick to the plan; just make sure it's not too sweet.

All the fiber is gone—I often see blender and smoothie advertisements telling people that ALL the fiber has been removed from juices. This is NOT accurate. It only takes a quick look at any juice to see that there is fiber still present in the juice but it's mostly the soluble kind. Soluble fiber absorbs water like a sponge; soluble fiber is the most important type for the regulation of sugar absorption. It slows the transit of food through the intestines and it feeds the good bacteria in our bowels to ensure a healthy colon. Soluble fibers include pectins, gums, and mucilage. All the soluble fiber remains in the juice.

Nutrients are lost in the pulp—There is some loss of nutrients in the pulp, but many of the nutrients are not bound to the fiber. The more efficient your juicer is and the drier the pulp, the more juice and nutrients you will get in your juice. From an independent source, it was demonstrated that if you use an average juicer, the juice contains 70% of the nutrients. Since you can consume approximately 4–6 times as many fruits and vegetables if you drink them in juice form, even with a 30% loss, your nutrient intake will still increase greatly.

Therefore, when consuming juice as a meal, you are ingesting 280–420% more nutrients than if you blended or ate it whole. Furthermore, with blending, you can use only some vegetables as others can be unpalatable in a blend. Make a carrot, apple, ginger, broccoli, and beet blend in a blender, and let me know how that goes! By the time you add ALL that water so you can actually drink it, it may take you all day to get through it. You also need to add more fruit to blends to make them more palatable.

You can clearly see many of the nutrients. The pigments found in fruits and vegetables are evident to the eye. Darkly colored fruits and vegetables and bright pigments all indicate a high level of nutrients. Take a look at a glass of juice versus a smoothie and you can soon see which one is more nutrient dense.

chapter 3. The 7-Day ACV Cleanse Plan

Your 7-Day Schedule

	DAY 1	DAY 2	DAY 3
On Rising	Morning Drink	Morning Drink	Morning Drink
Breakfast	Grapefruit Cleanser Juice	Grapefruit Cleanser Juice	Spiced Carrot Cake Juice
Morning Snack	Green Tea or Herbal tea Green Apple	Green Tea or Herbal tea Pear	Green Tea or Herbal tea 1 cup of Strawberries
Lunch	Antioxidant Beet Blend Vegetable Munch (optional) 1 Tb. of ACV	Energizing Red Juice Vegetable Munch (optional) 1 Tb. of ACV	Berry Green Blend Spiced Fries (½ recipe) (optional) 1 Tb. of ACV
Afternoon Snack	Green Cleanse Juice	Energizing Red Juice	Green Cleanse Juice
Dinner	Cauliflower Soup and/or Rainbow Salad with ACV Vinaigrette 1 Tb. of ACV	Cooling Cucumber Gazpacho and/or Spiced Fries 1 Tb. of ACV	Cauliflower Soup (½ recipe) and/or Arugula & Fennel Salad with Goddess Dressing 1 Tb. of ACV
Supper	Herbal Tea	Herbal Tea	Herbal Tea

DAY 4	DAY 5	DAY 6	DAY 7
Morning Drink	Morning Drink	Morning Drink	Morning Drink
Ginger Citrus Juice	Slim Grin Juice	Green Cleanse Juice	Ginger Citrus Juice
Green Tea or Herbal tea 1 slice of Pineapple	Green Tea or Herbal tea ½ cup of Blueberries	Green Tea or Herbal tea Pear	Green Tea or Herbal tea ½ cup of Blueberries
Green Cleanse Juice Vegetable Munch (optional) 1 Tb. of ACV	Antioxidant Beet Blend Roasted Broccoli (½ recipe) (optional) 1 Tb. of ACV	Grapefruit Cleanser Juice Green Bean Chips (optional) 1 Tb. of ACV	Golden Lime Blend Caprese Salad (optional) 1 Tb. of ACV
Spiced Carrot Cake Juice	Slim Grin Juice	Spicy Tomato Juice	Energizing Red Juice
Rainbow Salad with ACV Vinaigrette and/or Roasted Broccoli 1 Tb. of ACV	Cream of Greens Soup and/or Caprese Salad 1 Tb. of ACV	Cream of Greens Soup and/or Green Bean Chips (½ recipe) 1 Tb. of ACV	Arugula & Fennel Salad with Goddess Dressing and/or 1 Sliced Apple 1 Tb. of ACV
Herbal Tea	Herbal Tea	Herbal Tea	Herbal Tea

WATER: Drink 16 oz. of water in between each meal and snack (4 times daily) to enhance weight loss.

Note: Drink a supplement of 1 tablespoon of ACV when indicated. To be effective, ACV must be consumed within the 30 minutes before or after the meal.

Make sure you are drinking enough water in between meals to keep your energy levels up and to support the process of losing weight.

Shopping List for the Entire 7 Days

Fruit

- Apples • 18
- Avocado • 3
- Blueberries • 2 cups
- Cherries • 2 cups
- Grapefruit, Ruby • 5
- Lemons • 10
- Limes • 5
- Pears • 2
- Pineapple • 2 medium (9 thick slices)
- Strawberries • 1½ cup

Vegetables

- Arugula • 2 handfuls
- Beet leaves • 2 handfuls
- Beets • 8 (medium)
- Broccoli • 2 heads
- Carrots • 18
- Cauliflower • ½ head
- Celery • 4-5 bunches (36 stems)
- Chard • 2-3 bunches (24 leaves)
- Cucumbers • 11
- Fennel • 1
- Green beans • 2 handfuls
- Kale • 3 bunches (26 leaves)
- Kale leaves, baby • 2 handfuls
- Leeks • 2
- Parsnips • 2
- Red onions • 2
- Red bell pepper • 1
- Romaine lettuce • 1 bunch (8 leaves)
- Scallions • 9 scallions
- Spinach • 2 bunches
- Tomatoes • 5
- Tomatoes, cherry • 1 cup
- Zucchini (summer squash) • 1

Other

- Apple cider vinegar • 16 ounces
- Chia seeds
- Chili powder (optional)
- Cinnamon
- Coconut oil
- Coconut water • 4 cups
- Cumin
- Fresh basil • 2 handfuls
- Fresh chili • 6 small (optional)
- Fresh ginger • 10 inches
- Garlic • 6 cloves
- Green olives • 12

- Herbal tea blends
- Honey/stevia
- Nutmeg
- Olive oil
- Oregano, dried (optional)
- Paprika (optional)
- Fresh parsley • 3 bunches
- Vegetable stock (additive-free organic or homemade) • 32 ounces

Recipes for the Cleanse

Remember to always wash your produce and soak your vegetables in ACV (a natural cleaning agent). Chop your fruits and vegetables according to the size of your juicer. If you want to prepare ahead of time, then chopping and prepping your produce can be helpful.

You can also make and store your juices ahead of time. If you plan to drink them within 48 hours, then storing them in an airtight glass jar filled up to the top and stored at the back of the fridge will keep many of the nutrients intact. If you plan to drink them beyond 48 hours, then I suggest freezing them. Remember to leave a little room at the top of the jar to allow for expansion. There can be some small nutrient losses when you prepare ahead. But it's more important that you are able to stick with the ACV Cleanse. A juice that has 10% nutrient loss is better than NO juice at all.

Serving juice with ice can improve the palatability. Some people ask me if they can warm them in cooler weather, and the answer is yes, slightly. Adding warming spices can also assist in the coldness that some people may not enjoy. Ginger, turmeric, cinnamon, nutmeg, and chili all add warmth to the juices.

Remember to note that a juice or smoothie serving is approximately 2 cups (16 oz.).

The 7-Day ACV Cleanse Recipes

This collection of ACV recipes covers all the bases for your 7-Day Cleanse. Any of the ACV blended drinks in the first section can be used as your "Morning Drink" or in place of drinking pure ACV. If you find yourself wanting other options, check out the Alternative Recipes to find great substitutes.

Morning
Drink

To take on rising, this is a great hydrating and energizing beverage that includes lemon and ACV, giving you the best start to your day. Drink each morning for improved digestion, blood sugar levels and liver support, along with the other myriad health benefits that both the lemon and ACV have to offer. **Note:** The honey can reduce the acidity of the ACV and make it more palatable.

½ fresh lemon (juiced)

1 tablespoon of apple cider vinegar

1 cup of warm or hot water

Grated fresh ginger (optional)

1 teaspoon of honey or stevia (optional)

Steep for 5 minutes, then strain and drink.

Amount Per Serving • % Daily Value

Serving Size 291g | Calories 40 | Calories from Fat 2 | Total Fat 0.2g • 0% | Trans Fat 0g | Cholesterol 0mg • 0% | Sodium 9mg • 0% | Potassium 85mg • 2% | Total Carbohydrates 10.1g • 3% | Dietary Fiber 1.1g • 4% | Sugars 6.6g | Protein 0.5g | Vitamin A 0% | Vitamin C 27% | Calcium 2% | Iron 3%

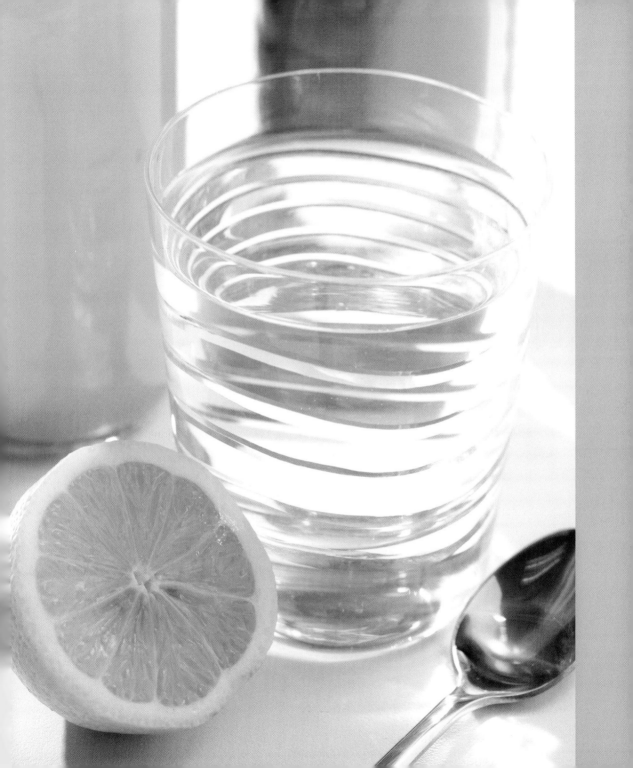

ACV Drinks

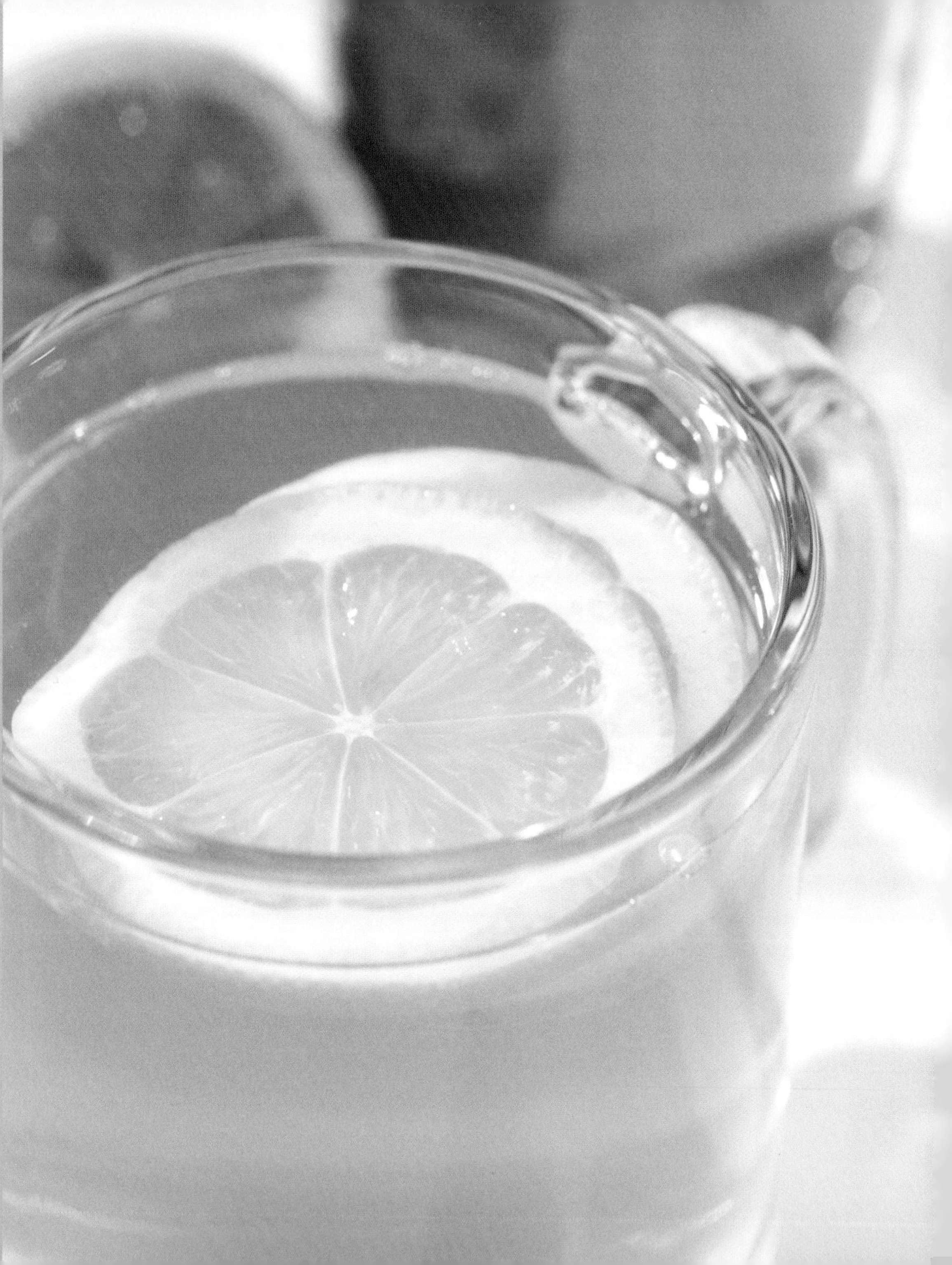

Green Tea
with ACV

Green tea is a natural energizer due to its stimulating properties. The benefits of green tea are potentiated by the phytonutrient compounds naturally present in both the lemon and the ACV. This is a great hot beverage to enjoy in the mornings.

1 organic green tea bag

1 teaspoon of apple cider vinegar

1 tablespoon of lemon juice

1 cup of hot water

1 teaspoon of honey or stevia (optional)

Leave to steep in cup and remove tea bag after 5 minutes.

Amount Per Serving • % Daily Value

Serving Size 22g | Calories 5 | Calories from Fat 1 | Total Fat 0.1g • 0% | Trans Fat 0g | Cholesterol 0mg • 0% | Sodium 3mg • 0% | Potassium 73mg • 2% | Total Carbohydrates 0.4g • 0% | Protein 0.1g | Vitamin A 0% | Vitamin C 12% | Calcium 0% | Iron 0%

Sparkling
ACV Water ....

This is a great alternative to soda drinks. If you like a few bubbles, adding in ACV gives sparkling water great flavor while being a nice way to enjoy the health benefits of ACV. This is one of my personal favorites.

1 cup of club soda or sparkling mineral water
1 tablespoon of apple cider vinegar
1 teaspoon of honey or stevia (optional)

Mix together for a very refreshing drink to consume as an alternative to soda. This can be a fun way to consume your ACV with your dinner.

Amount Per Serving • % Daily Value

Serving Size 255g | Calories 14 | Calories from Fat 0 | Total Fat 0.0g • 0% | Trans Fat 0g | Cholesterol 0mg • 0% | Sodium 51mg • 2% | Potassium 18mg • 1% | Total Carbohydrates 3.0g • 1% | Sugars 2.9g | Protein 0.0g | Vitamin A 0% | Vitamin C 0% | Calcium 1% | Iron 0%

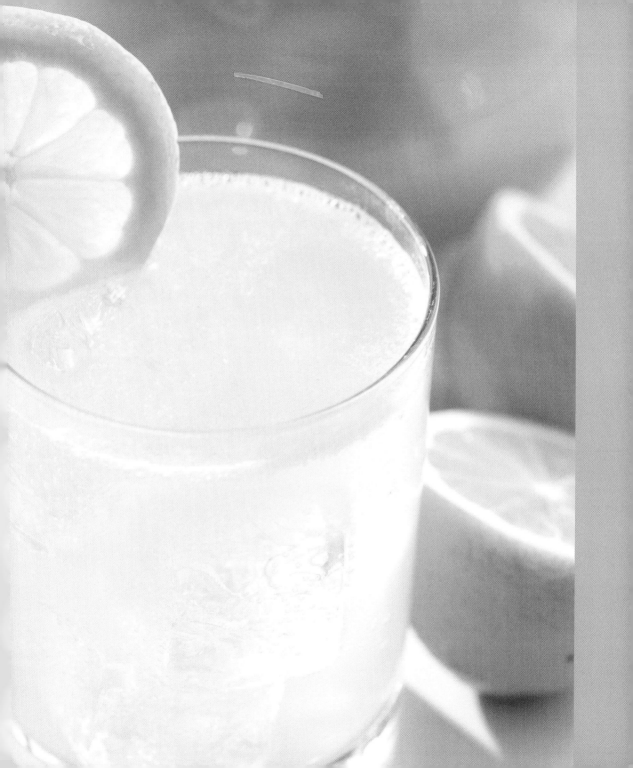

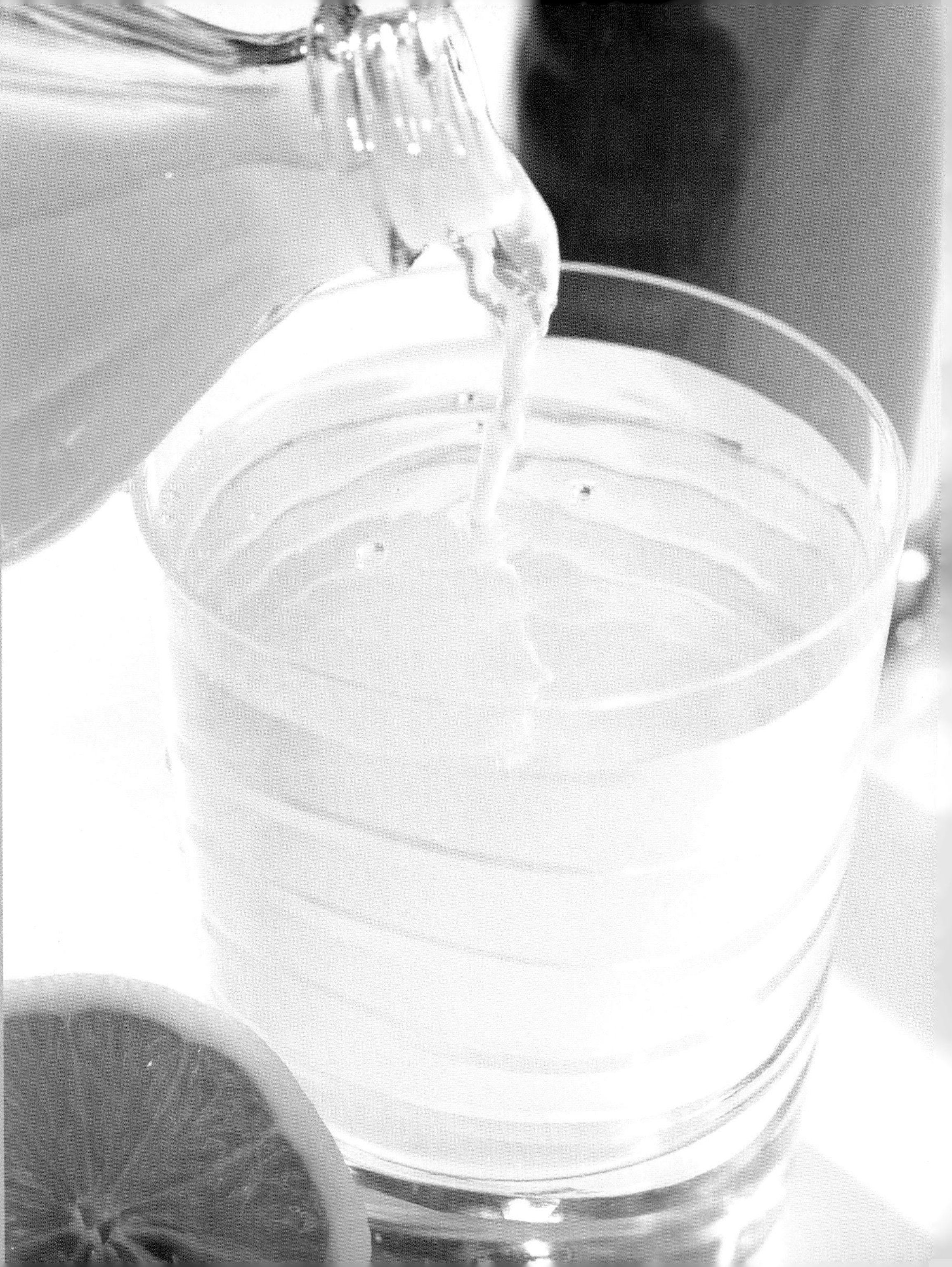

Metabolic
ACV Drink

This is a drink that is specifically formulated to help stimulate the metabolism and support fat burning and blood sugar control. This drink may not be for everyone due to the cayenne pepper but it certainly can help support the process of weight control.

1 cup of water

1 tablespoon of apple cider vinegar

1 tablespoon of lemon juice

½ teaspoon of cinnamon

1 dash of cayenne pepper (optional)

Stevia or honey to taste (optional)

1 teaspoon of grated ginger (optional)

Stir all ingredients together.

Amount Per Serving • % Daily Value

Serving Size 276g | Calories 32 | Calories from Fat 2 | Total Fat 0.2g • 0% | Trans Fat 0g | Cholesterol 0mg • 0% | Sodium 11mg • 0% | Potassium 45mg • 1% | Total Carbohydrates 7.3g • 2% | Dietary Fiber 0.7g • 3% | Sugars 6.2g | Protein 0.2g | Vitamin A 2% | Vitamin C 12% | Calcium 2% | Iron 1%

ACV Juices

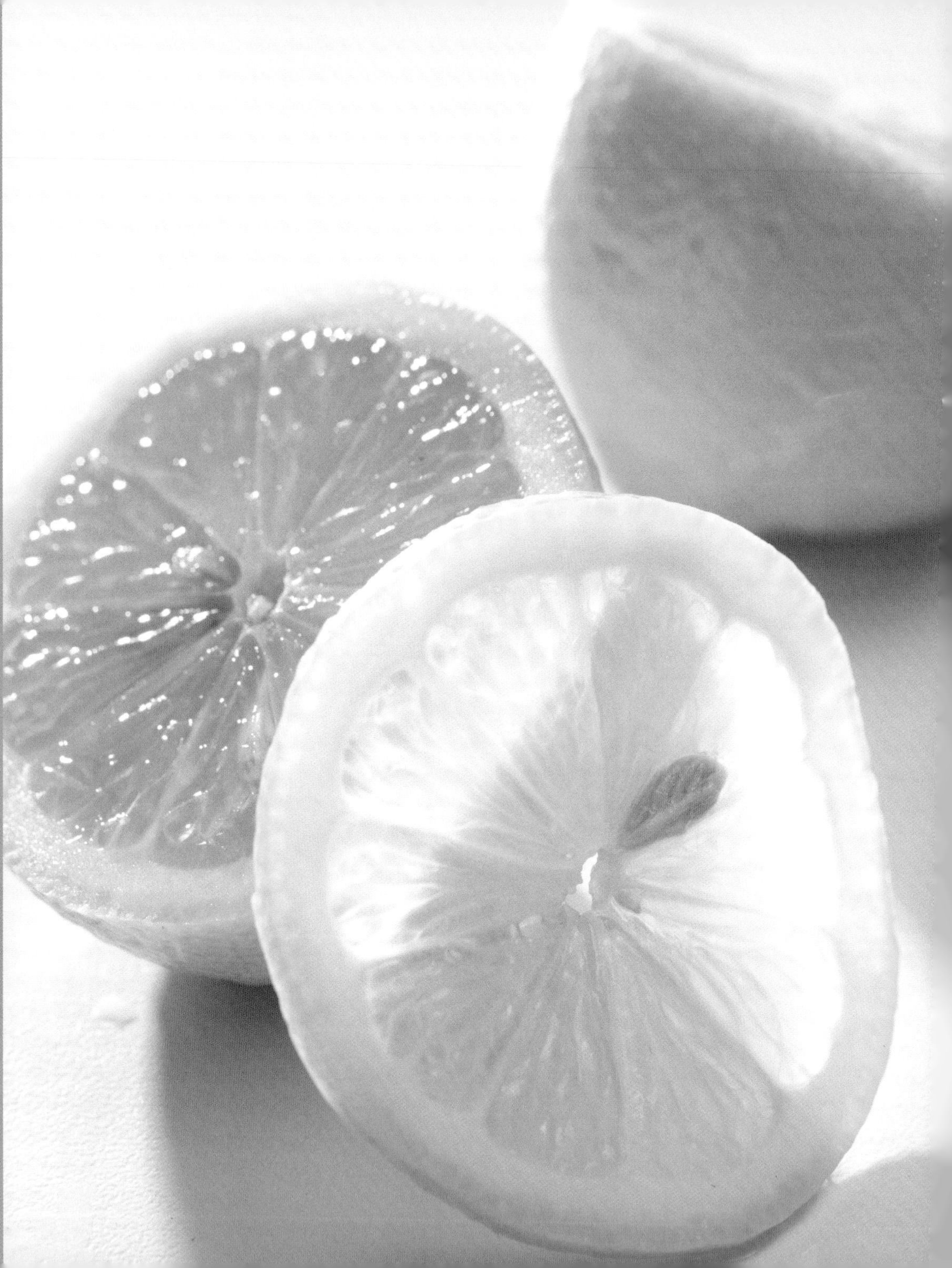

Grapefruit
Cleanser Juice

Including the consumption of grapefruit helps to improve weight control, and reduces the risk of obesity, diabetes, and heart disease while promoting a healthy complexion and increased energy. This is a great juice to include for the many nutrients and weight-loss support. When taking medications, it is best to check with your doctor about grapefruit, as it can be contra-indicated.

1 ruby grapefruit, peeled
1 lemon
4 Swiss chard leaves
2 carrots

Wash, chop, and juice.

16 oz. = 1 serving | Amount Per Serving • % Daily Value (Juiced)

Serving Size 502g | Calories 104 | Calories from Fat 7.4 | Total Fat 0.82g• 2.3% | Saturated Fat 0.118g• 0.6% | Trans Fat 0g | Cholesterol 0mg | Sodium 341mg • 22.7% | Potassium 1161mg • 24.7% | Total Carbohydrates 32.7g • 25.2% | Dietary Fiber 1.2g • 3.2% | Sugars 19.2g | Protein 4.9g | Vitamin A 132.2% | Vitamin C 131.6% | Calcium 13.2% | Iron 39.3%

Green Cleanse
Juice

This is a cleansing high-nutrient juice that contains high amounts of iron, magnesium, calcium (253 mg), potassium, vitamin A, vitamin C, vitamin K, B vitamins and protein at 7 g per serving. These fruits and vegetables are also supportive of improved liver function, energy, and digestion.

4 kale leaves
2 apples
1 cucumber
1 lime
4 celery sticks
1 inch of ginger

Wash, chop, and juice.

16 oz. = 1 serving | Amount Per Serving • % Daily Value (Juiced)

Serving Size 914 g | Calories 191 | Calories from Fat 16.1 | Total Fat 1.79 g • 5.1% | Saturated Fat 0.282 g • 1.4% | Trans Fat 0 g | Cholesterol 0 mg | Sodium 83 mg • 5.5% | Potassium 1324 mg • 28.2% | Total Carbohydrate 58.4 g • 44.9% | Dietary Fiber 1.8 g • 4.7% | Sugars 33.3 g | Protein 6.94 g | Vitamin A 56.9% | Vitamin C 143.6% | Calcium 22.9% | Iron 34%

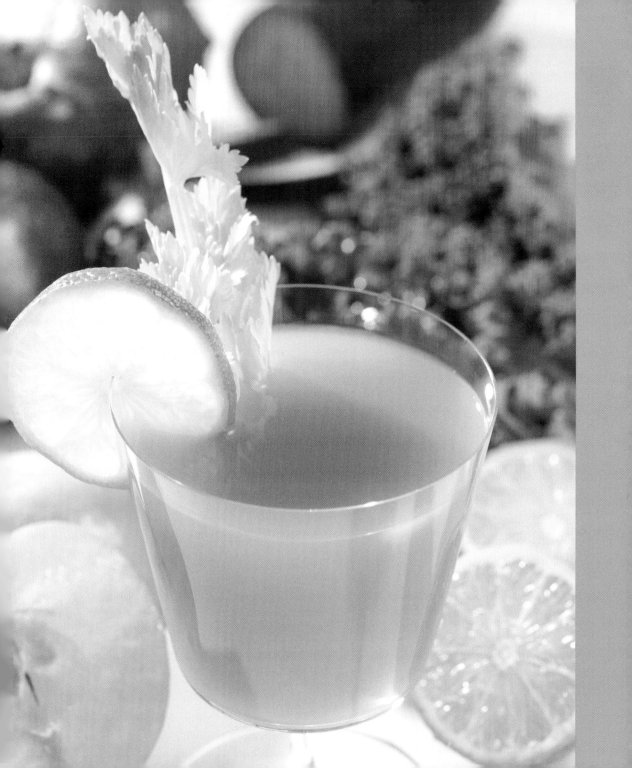

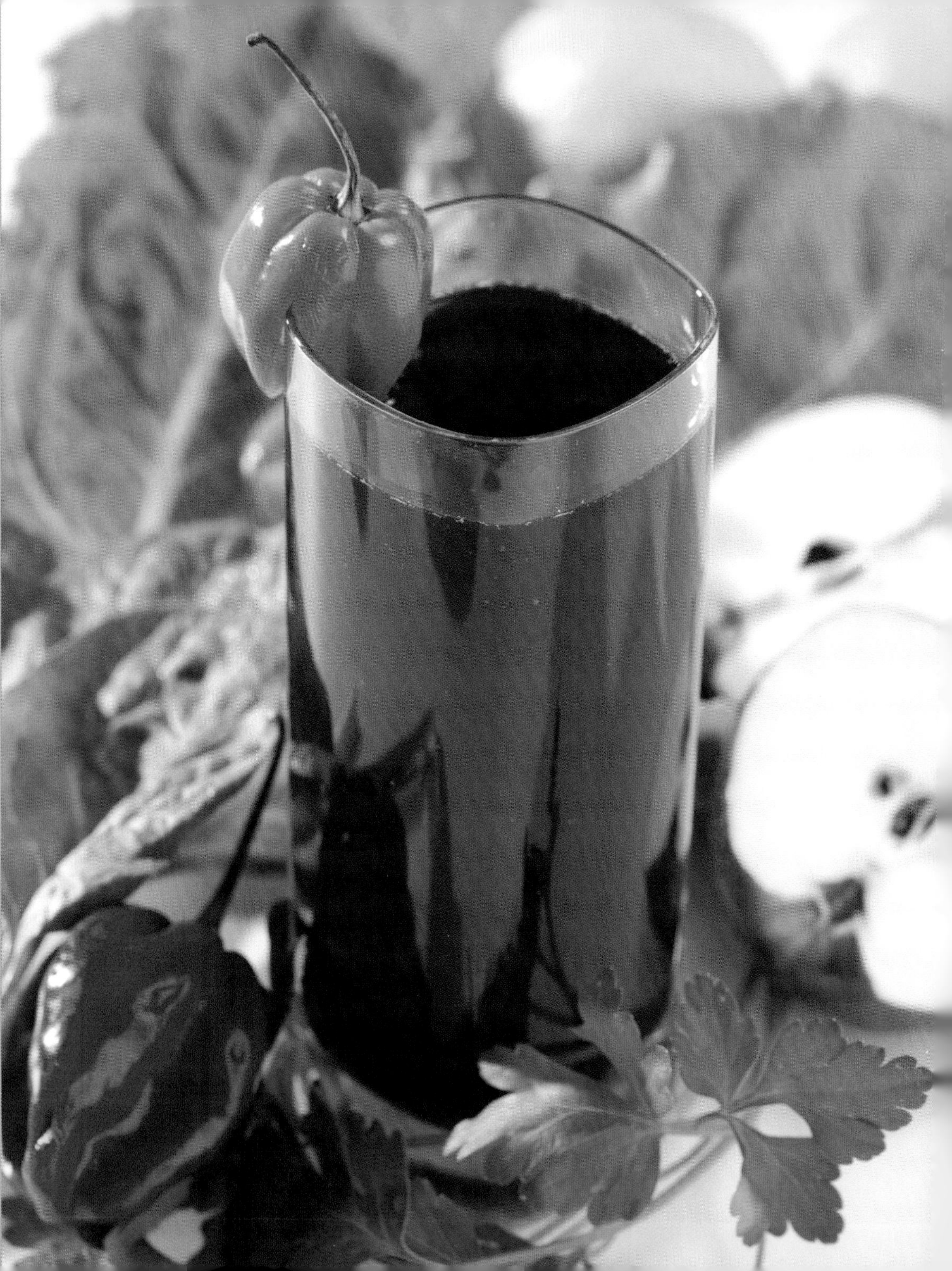

Energizing
Red Juice

Beets and chard are both high in natural nitric oxide, which supports improved energy and exercise performance. This is a great juice for muscle aches and pains and to give you that extra pep-me-up for your day. This is a high-nutrient juice to include in the plan.

2 beets

4 Swiss chard leaves (and stems)

½ bunch of spinach

1 apple

1 handful of parsley

1 lemon

1 small chili (optional)

Wash, chop, and juice.

16 oz. = 1 serving | Amount Per Serving • % Daily Value (Juiced)

Serving Size 819g | Calories 187 | Calories from Fat 15.7 | Total Fat 1.74g • 5% | Saturated Fat 0.273g • 1.4% | Trans Fat 0g | Cholesterol 0mg | Sodium 581mg • 38.7% | Potassium 2443mg • 52% | Total Carbohydrate 56.8g • 43.7% | Dietary Fiber 2.5g • 6.6% | Sugars 33.01g | Protein 11.41g | Vitamin A 120.1% | Vitamin C 152.4% | Calcium 28.3% | Iron 121.4%

Spiced Carrot Cake Juice ....

This is an enjoyable dessert-style juice that is packed full of nutrients and is high in carotenoids, particularly beta-carotene. This is a delicious, easy juice to consume with the added benefits of the cinnamon, including blood sugar control and appetite regulation.

3 large carrots
2 apples
3 celery sticks
1 inch of fresh ginger
1 pinch of cinnamon
1 tiny pinch of nutmeg

Wash, chop, and juice.

16 oz. = 1 serving | Amount Per Serving • % Daily Value (Juiced)

Serving Size 602g | Calories 169 | Calories from Fat 8.9 | Total Fat 0.99g • 2.83% | Saturated Fat 0.2g • 0.9% | Trans Fat 0g | Cholesterol 0mg | Sodium 173mg • 11.5% | Potassium 1053mg • 22.4% | Total Carbohydrate 52.9g • 40.7% | Dietary Fiber 1.7g • 4.5% | Sugars 34.41g | Protein 2.76g | Vitamin A 141.1% | Vitamin C 22.6% | Calcium 9.9% | Iron 12%

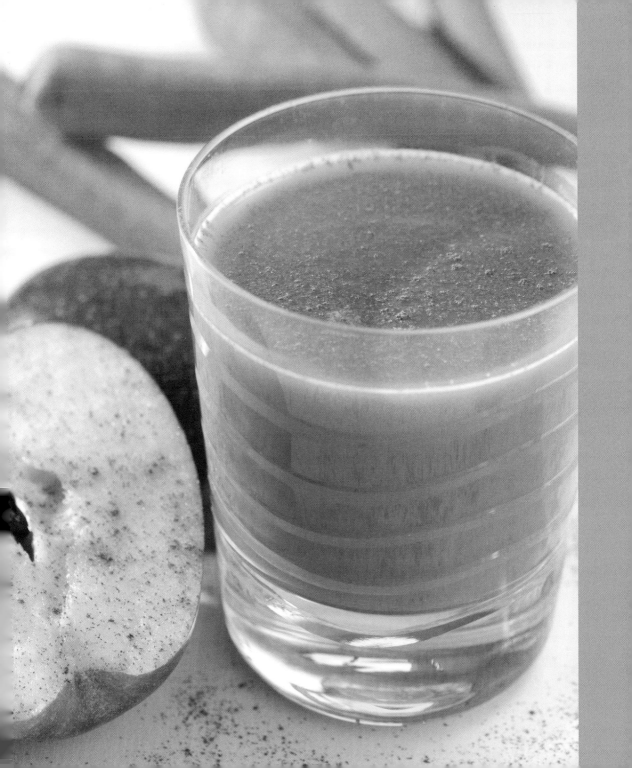

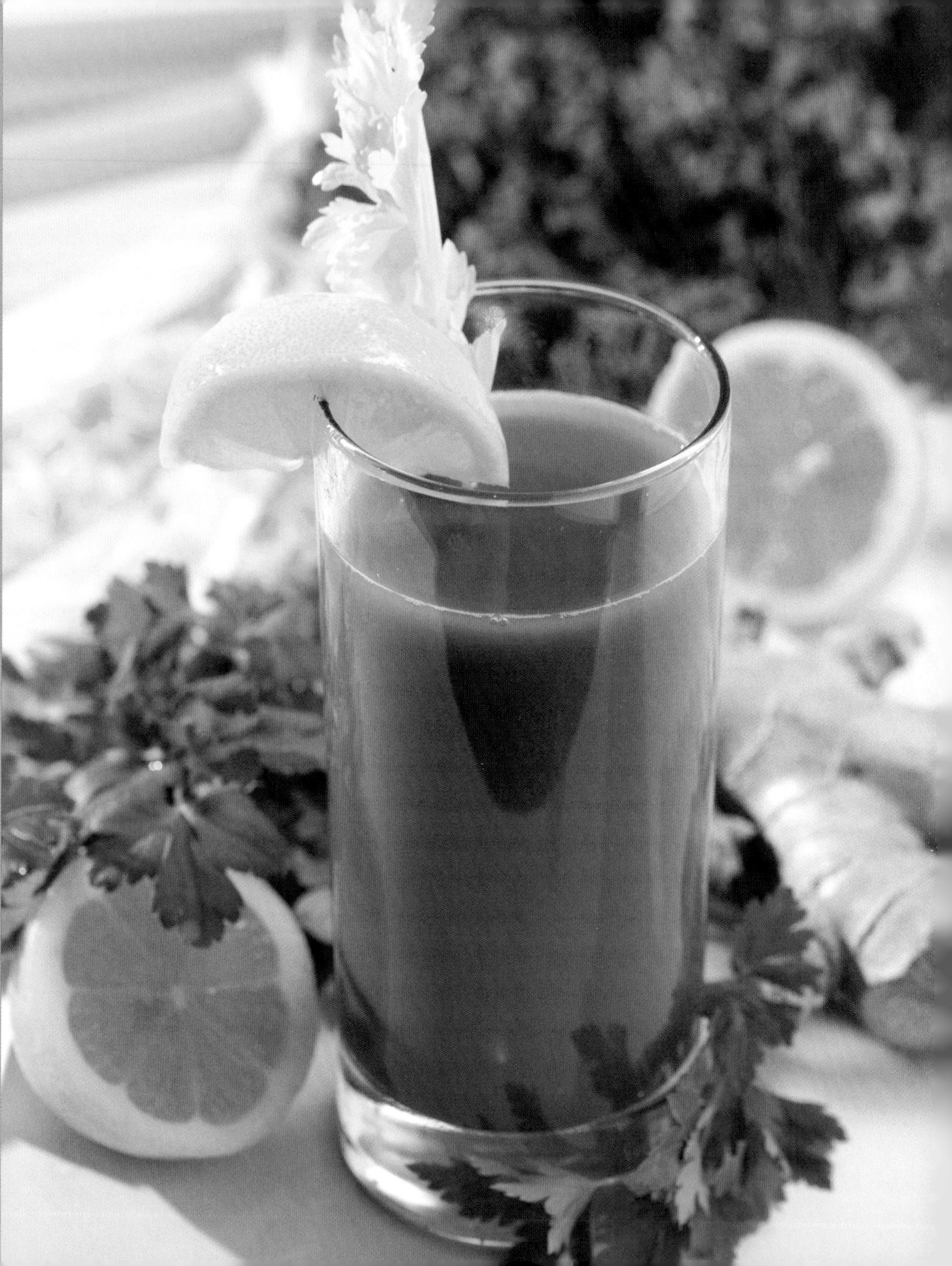

Slim **Grin**
Juice

This is a light green juice with the added benefit of the pineapples. Pineapples supply brome-lain, which helps to reduce inflammation and support the healing of injured tissue and osteo-arthritis. This juice is also high in vitamin C, potassium, magnesium, protein (6 g), vitamin A, B vitamins, and vitamin K.

2 slices of pineapple, peeled

4 kale leaves

2 celery stalks

4 large leaves of romaine lettuce

1 handful of flat parsley

1 lemon

1 inch of fresh ginger

1 chili

Wash, chop, and juice.

16 oz. = 1 serving | Amount Per Serving • % Daily Value (Juiced)

Serving Size 499g | Calories 131 | Calories from Fat 17.1 | Total Fat 1.9g • 5.4% | Saturated Fat 0.2g • 1.1% | Trans Fat 0g | Cholesterol 0mg | Sodium 83mg • 5.5% | Potassium 1290mg • 27.5% | Total Carbohydrate 38.3g • 29.4% | Dietary Fiber 1.5g • 4% | Sugars 18.3g | Protein 8.1g | Vitamin A 106.7% | Vitamin C 277.9% | Calcium 25.4% | Iron 4.9862.3%

Ginger
Citrus Juice

This is a very refreshing juice that contains the benefits of the grapefruit, which is great for blood sugar regulation and weight loss and has a high vitamin C content. The pineapple offers excellent anti-inflammatory benefits along with the ginger, which is an excellent digestive spice.

1 thick slice of pineapple, peeled
1 grapefruit, peeled
1 lemon
4 celery sticks
1 inch of fresh ginger

Wash, chop, and juice.

16 oz. = 1 serving | Amount Per Serving • % Daily Value (Juiced)

Serving Size 342g | Calories 123 | Calories from Fat 5.7 | Total Fat 0.6g • 1.8% | Saturated Fat 0.1g • 0.5% | Trans Fat 0g | Cholesterol 0mg | Sodium 41mg • 2.7% | Potassium 642mg • 13.7% | Total Carbohydrate 37.57g • 28.9% | Dietary Fiber 0.9g • 2.4% | Sugars 25.83g | Protein 2.84g | Vitamin A 10.7% | Vitamin C 143.1% | Calcium 7.1% | Iron 12.3%

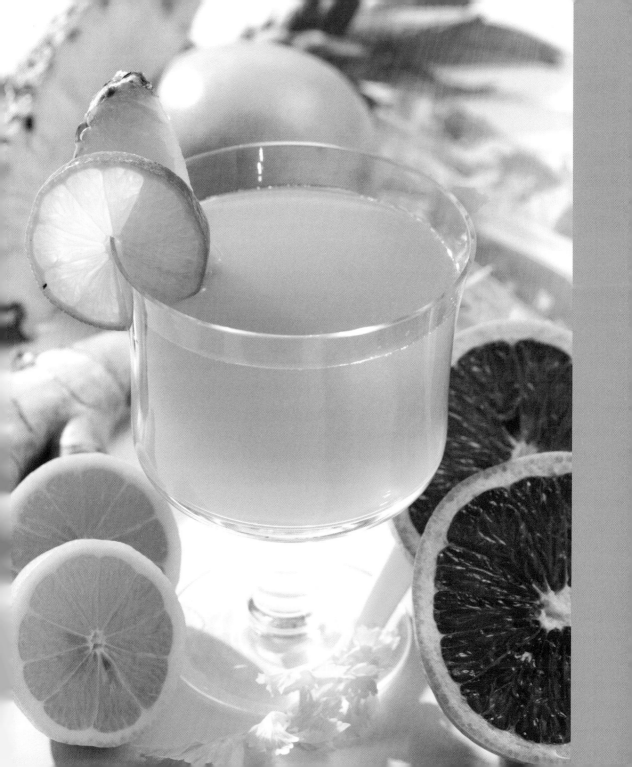

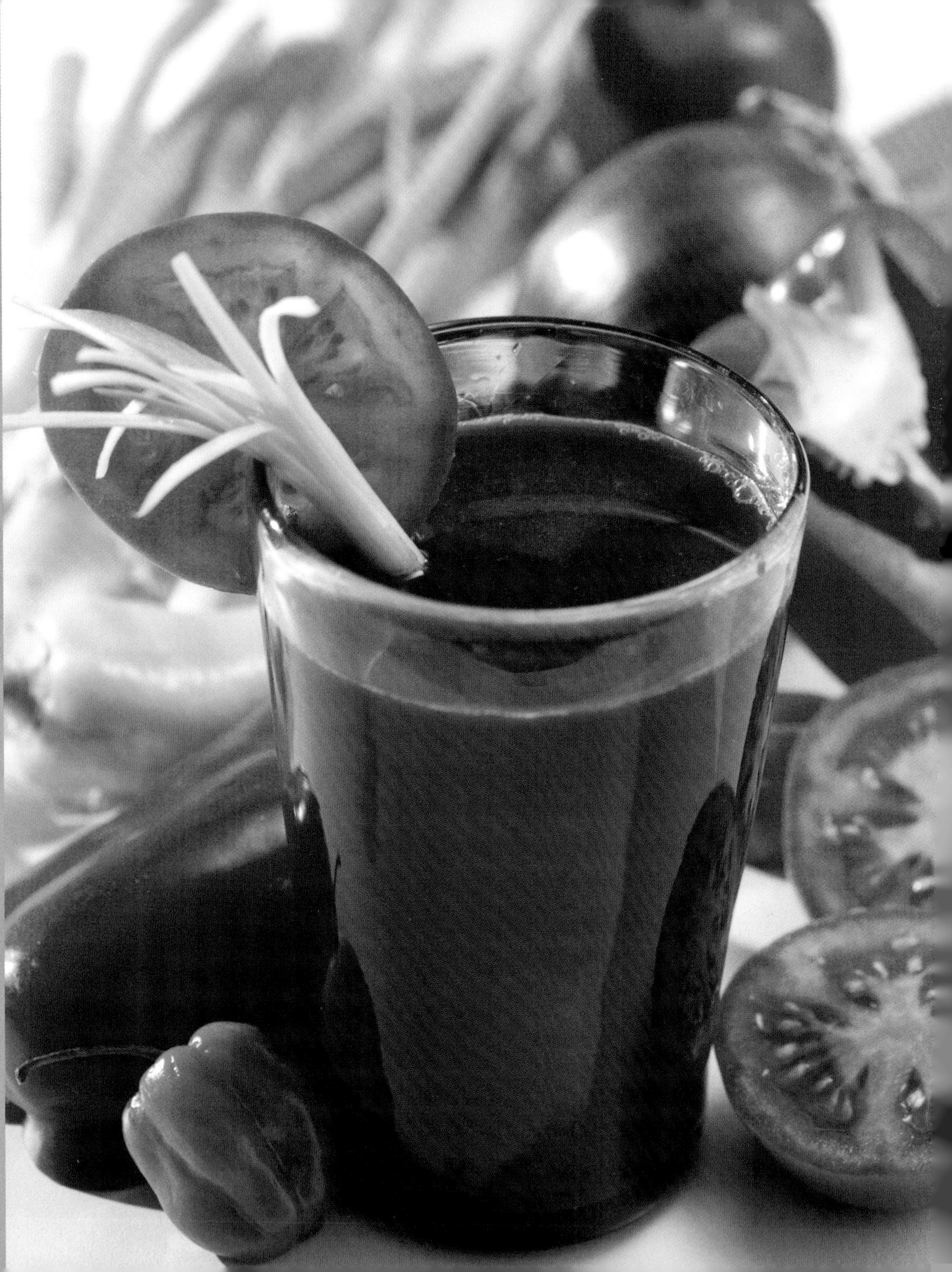

Spicy
Tomato Juice

This is a great spicy and savory juice. If you love tomato soup and savory juices, such as the well-known V8, then you will love this. Tomatoes contain an important antioxidant called lycopene, which supports heart health, skin health, and prostate health for men.

3 large tomatoes

1 celery stick

2 carrots

1 red bell pepper

¼ red onion

1–2 fresh chilis (optional)

2 scallions

Wash, chop, and juice.

16 oz. = 1 serving | Amount Per Serving • % Daily Value (Juiced)

Serving Size 701g | Calories 106 | Calories from Fat 11.3 | Total Fat 1.3g • 3.6% | Saturated Fat 0.2g • 0.9% | Trans Fat 0g | Cholesterol 0mg | Sodium 91mg • 6.1% | Potassium 1495mg • 31.8% | Total Carbohydrates 30.3g • 23.3% | Dietary Fiber 1.3g • 3.4% | Sugars 18.5g | Protein 5.3g | Vitamin A 110.7% | Vitamin C 158.9% | Calcium 8.5% | Iron 22.4%

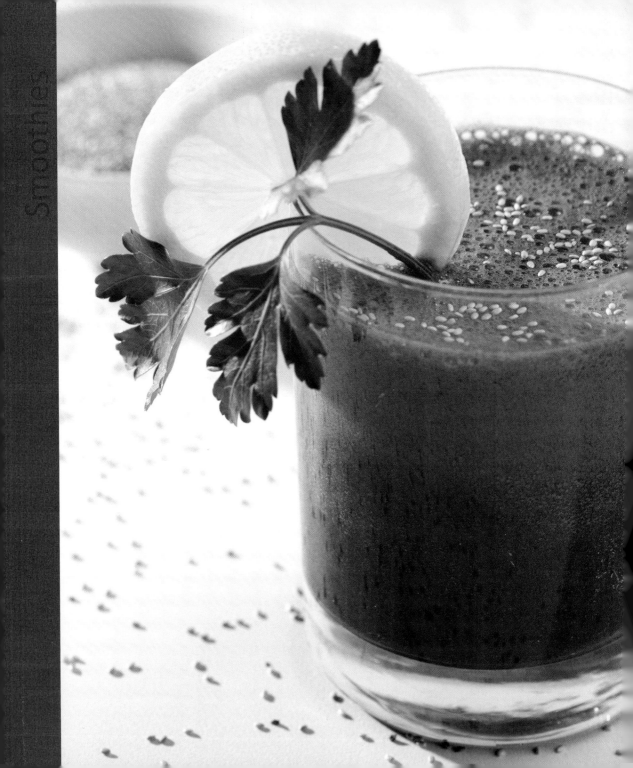

Antioxidant
Beet Blend

This is a great sweet-but-not-too-sweet smoothie recipe that offers the benefits of the beet fiber combined with the very high antioxidant-containing cherries. This is an easy, delicious, and filling smoothie to enjoy for your lunch meal. **Note:** Beets have a strong flavor. I suggest starting with less than the recommended amount and tasting it as you go. The cherries and coconut water sweeten this smoothie naturally.

1 cup of cherries (fresh or frozen)
¼ small beet
Handful of baby spinach leaves
1 cup of coconut water
1 handful of ice
1 tablespoon of chia seeds
1 teaspoon of honey or stevia to taste (optional)

Wash, chop, and blend.

1 serving | Amount Per Serving • % Daily Value

Serving Size 487g | Calories 247 | Calories from Fat 24 | Total Fat 2.7g • 4% | Trans Fat 0g | Cholesterol 0mg • 0% | Sodium 88mg • 4% | Potassium 834mg • 24% | Total Carbohydrates 56.7g • 19% | Dietary Fiber 4.3g • 17% | Sugars 24.3g | Protein 3.0g | Vitamin A 33% | Vitamin C 246% | Calcium 13% | Iron 9%

Berry
Green Blend

This is a simple and delicious smoothie recipe that includes the benefits of the leafy greens with the berries for their high antioxidant content. Studies show that berries and spinach are very beneficial in protecting the brain from oxidative damage and supporting a healthy memory.

1 cup of coconut water
Handful of spinach
½ small cucumber
½ celery stick
½ lemon (juiced, optional)
1 cup of blueberries (fresh or frozen)
Handful of ice as desired
1 tablespoon of chia seeds

Wash, chop, and blend.

1 serving | Amount Per Serving • % Daily Value

Serving Size 468g | Calories 210 | Calories from Fat 30 | Total Fat 3.4g • 5% | Trans Fat 0g | Cholesterol 0mg • 0% | Sodium 57mg • 2% | Potassium 1021mg • 29% | Total Carbohydrates 48.4g • 16% | Dietary Fiber 8.2g • 33% | Sugars 33.0g | Protein 4.5g | Vitamin A 33% | Vitamin C 220% | Calcium 18% | Iron 24%

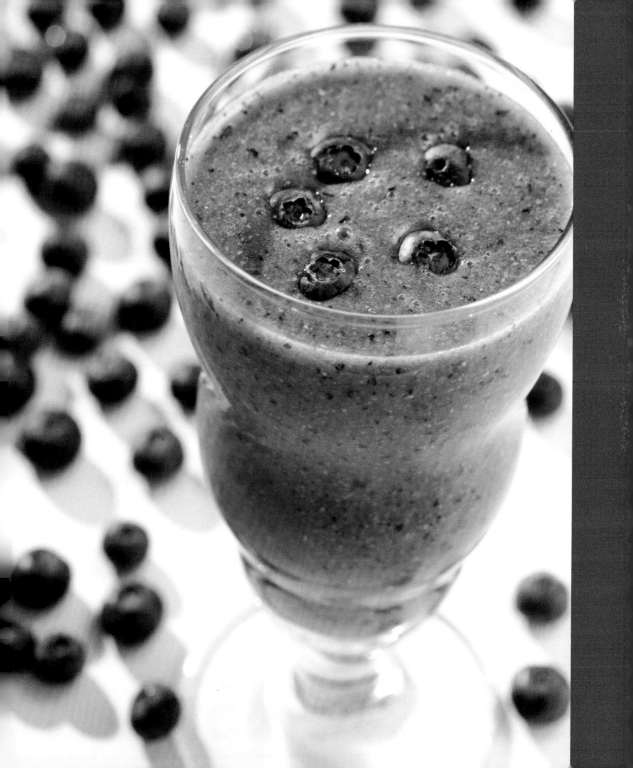

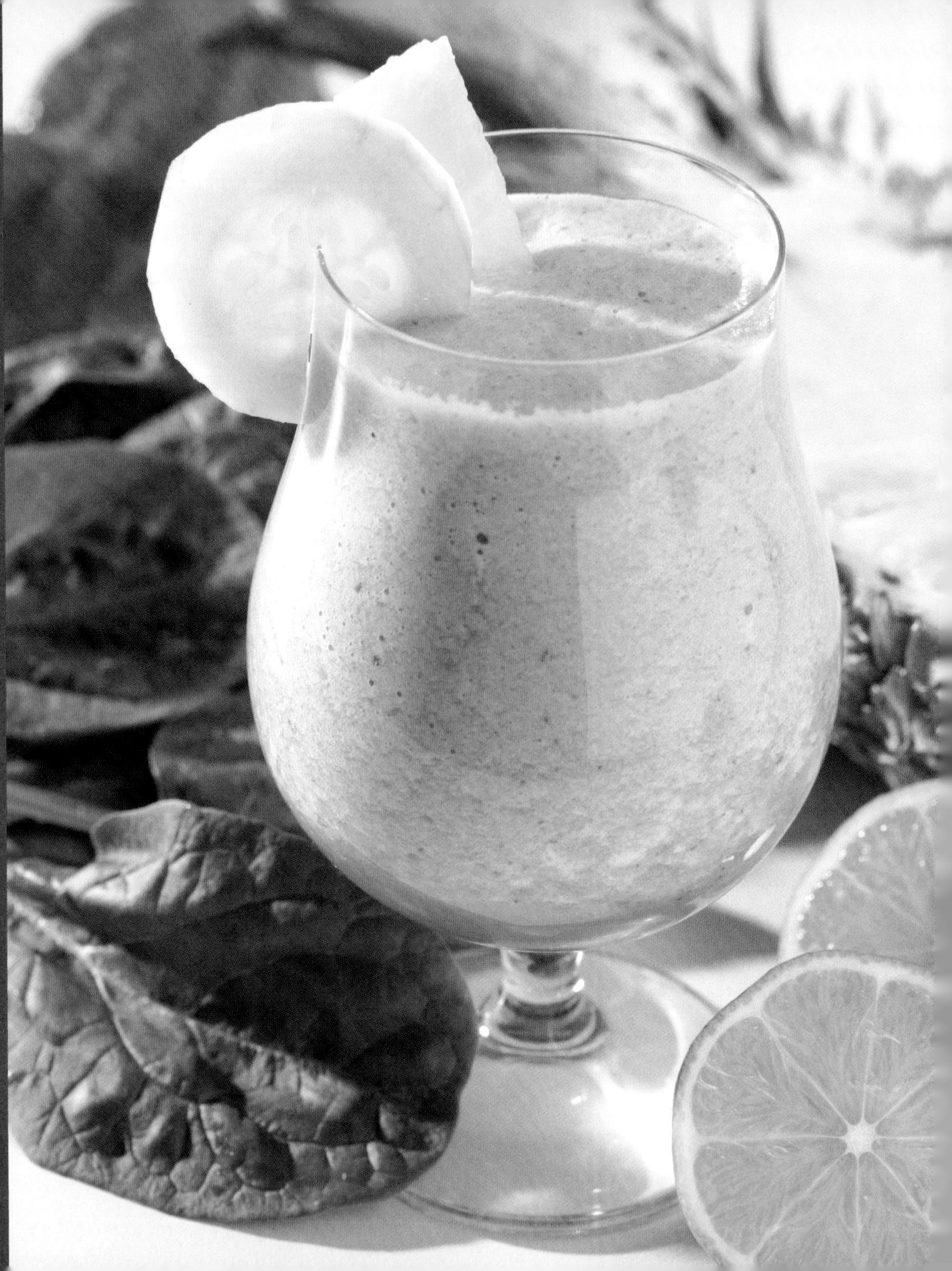

Golden Pine
Lime Blend

This is a light and tangy smoothie that is high in fiber, vitamin C, and phytonutrients. This is a simple and filling smoothie to enjoy as a meal to enhance weight loss and feelings of fullness.

1 cup of coconut water

1 thick slice of pineapple

Juice of 1 lime

1 handful of baby spinach leaves

½ cucumber

1 large handful of ice

Wash, chop, and blend.

1 serving | Amount Per Serving • % Daily Value

Serving Size 381g | Calories 131 | Calories from Fat 4 | Total Fat 0.4g • 1% | Trans Fat 0g | Cholesterol 0mg • 0% | Sodium 42mg • 2% | Potassium 888mg • 25% | Total Carbohydrates 34.5g • 12% | Dietary Fiber 3.5g • 14% | Sugars 24.0g | Protein 2.1g | Vitamin A 33% | Vitamin C 227% | Calcium 13% | Iron 12%

Vegetable
Munch

This is a light and easy snack to enjoy as an optional snack to help ease hunger and to enhance satisfaction on the plan. Filling easy snacks can be very helpful to support the success of the plan. **Note:** You can use any vegetable stick you fancy—peppers, asparagus, green beans, and broccoli florets also work well.

½ **avocado**

1 tablespoon apple cider vinegar

Salt and pepper (to taste)

1 celery stick

1 carrot

1 cucumber

Mash ½ avocado with 1 tablespoon ACV, salt, and pepper. Chop the celery, carrot, and cucumber into sticks.

2 servings | Amount Per Serving • % Daily Value

Serving Size 240g | Calories 139 | Calories from Fat 90 | Total Fat 10.0g • 15% | Saturated Fat 2.1g • 11% | Trans Fat 0g | Cholesterol 0mg • 0% | Sodium 34mg • 1% | Potassium 585mg • 17% | Total Carbohydrates 13.0g • 4% | Dietary Fiber 5.0g • 20% | Sugars 4.4g | Protein 2.2g | Vitamin A 107% | Vitamin C 19% | Calcium 4% | Iron 5%

Spiced
Fries

These are delicious and easy to make and will help anyone feel that you are not missing out on anything. These are a great compliment to the healthy main meal and to the lunch juice to help with satisfaction.

2 carrots, peeled and sliced into sticks

2 parsnips, sliced into thick sticks

1 tablespoon of olive oil or coconut oil

½ teaspoon of ground cumin

¼ teaspoon of ground chili powder (optional or to taste)

Salt and pepper (to taste)

Preheat oven to 425°F (220°C). Line a baking tray with parchment paper or aluminum foil. In a medium bowl combine and toss all the ingredients together. Transfer to the baking sheet, making sure no fries overlap. Bake for 20 to 25 minutes, tossing with tongs halfway through until lightly browned.

2 servings | Amount Per Serving • % Daily Value

Serving Size 170g | Calories 162 | Calories from Fat 67 | Total Fat 7.4g • 11% | Saturated Fat 1.1g • 5% | Trans Fat 0g | Cholesterol 0mg • 0% | Sodium 634mg • 26% | Potassium 579mg • 17% | Total Carbohydrates 24.2g • 8% | Dietary Fiber 6.4g • 26% | Sugars 7.8g | Protein 1.8g | Vitamin A 204% | Vitamin C 34% | Calcium 6% | Iron 6%

Roasted
Broccoli

This a new way to enjoy the many health benefits of broccoli. Roasting the broccoli helps to give it a lovely flavor that even the most avid broccoli hater can enjoy. Broccoli has the health benefits of improving and supporting natural liver detoxification and helps to protect against many types of cancer.

1 small head of broccoli, chopped into large bite-size pieces
2 garlic cloves, crushed
2 teaspoons of coconut oil or olive oil
Salt and pepper (to taste)

Preheat oven to 400°F (200°C) and line a baking tray with parchment paper. Toss ingredients together and arrange on the baking tray. Cook for 25–30 minutes.

2 servings | Amount Per Serving • % Daily Value

Serving Size 100g | Calories 75 | Calories from Fat 44 | Total Fat 4.9g • 7% | Saturated Fat 3.9g • 20% | Trans Fat 0g | Cholesterol 0mg • 0% | Sodium 612mg • 25% | Potassium 300mg • 9% | Total Carbohydrates 7.0g • 2% | Dietary Fiber 2.4g • 10% | Sugars 1.6g | Protein 2.7g | Vitamin A 11% | Vitamin C 137% | Calcium 5% | Iron 4%

Green Bean
Chips

Green beans are an easy and low-calorie snack to enjoy. They are high in nutrients and are filling and satisfying. Adding a little sea salt and spice makes a simple vegetable into a crispy delicious snack.

2 large handfuls of green beans
Salt and pepper (to taste)
Cayenne pepper or chili powder (optional)

Lightly blanch the green beans for 1 minute in boiling water, and then cool quickly. Season to taste.

2 servings | Amount Per Serving • % Daily Value

Serving Size 84g | Calories 26 | Calories from Fat 1 | Total Fat 0.1g • 0% | Cholesterol 0mg • 0% | Sodium 586mg • 24% | Potassium 173mg • 5% | Total Carbohydrates 5.9g • 2% | Dietary Fiber 2.8g • 11% | Sugars 1.2g | Protein 1.5g | Vitamin A 11% | Vitamin C 22% | Calcium 3% | Iron 5%

Soups

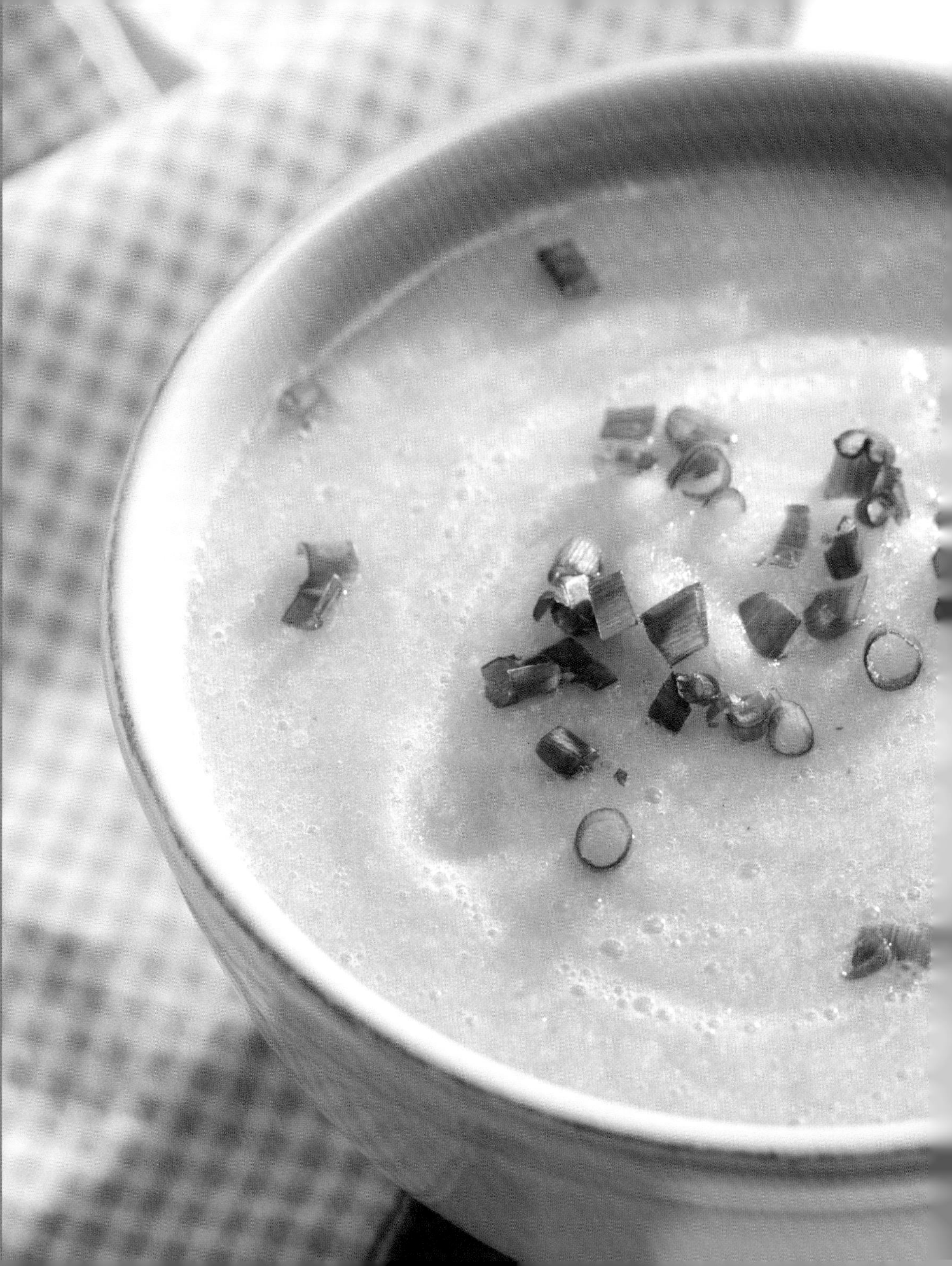

Cauliflower
Soup

This is one of my favorite easy, low-calorie, and high-nutrient soups to make to act as a satisfying and filling comfort meal. The anti-inflammatory cauliflower contains many phytonutrients that help to support liver detoxification.

½ large head of cauliflower, chopped

1 tablespoon of coconut oil or extra-virgin olive oil

2 garlic cloves, crushed

1 leek, white parts chopped

2–2 ½ cups of vegetable stock

Salt and pepper (to taste)

1 teaspoon of chives, chopped

Simmer the cauliflower in water for 15 minutes or until tender. In a saucepan, heat the oil over medium heat and sauté the garlic, leeks, and pinch of salt for about 3 minutes, until soft. Add the vegetable stock and simmer for about 5 minutes, or until it's hot; add in the drained cauliflower and blend it to form a thick consistency. Add more stock if it is too thick.

2 servings | Amount Per Serving • % Daily Value

Serving Size 397g | Calories 155 | Calories from Fat 78 | Total Fat 8.6g • 13% | Saturated Fat 1.4g • 7% | Cholesterol 0mg • 0% | Sodium 1384mg • 58% | Potassium 602mg • 17% | Total Carbohydrates 13.5g • 5% | Dietary Fiber 3.4g • 13% | Sugars 4.9g | Protein 7.7g | Vitamin A 15% | Vitamin C 88% | Calcium 6% | Iron 11%

Cooling **Cucumber** Gazpacho

This is a cooling, easy, and delicious soup that is truly satisfying and can be a great alternative to always drinking sweeter style smoothies or hot, savory soups. It is filling and very high in phytonutrient compounds to support good health and well-being.

½ avocado, peeled and cored

1 tablespoon of red onion

1 scallion, chopped

1 cup of water

¼ teaspoon of sea salt

½ cucumber, sliced

1 tablespoon of cold-pressed olive oil

1 tablespoon of lemon juice

1 tablespoon of apple cider vinegar

¼ teaspoon of cayenne

Pinch of paprika and chili powder

Salt and pepper (to taste)

Place all ingredients in the blender and process until smooth.

1 serving | Amount Per Serving • % Daily Value

Serving Size 323g | Calories 365 | Calories from Fat 306 | Total Fat 34.0g • 52% | Saturated Fat 6.3g • 32% | Trans Fat 0g | Cholesterol 0mg • 0% | Sodium 484mg • 20% | Potassium 804mg • 23% | Total Carbohydrates 16.8g • 6% | Dietary Fiber 8.3g • 33% | Sugars 4.2g | Protein 3.4g | Vitamin A 13% | Vitamin C 42% | Calcium 5% | Iron 7%

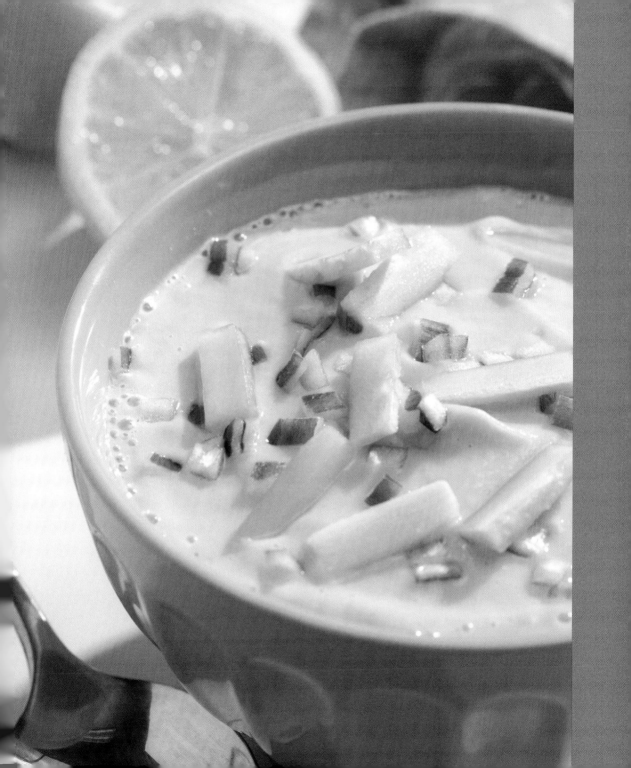

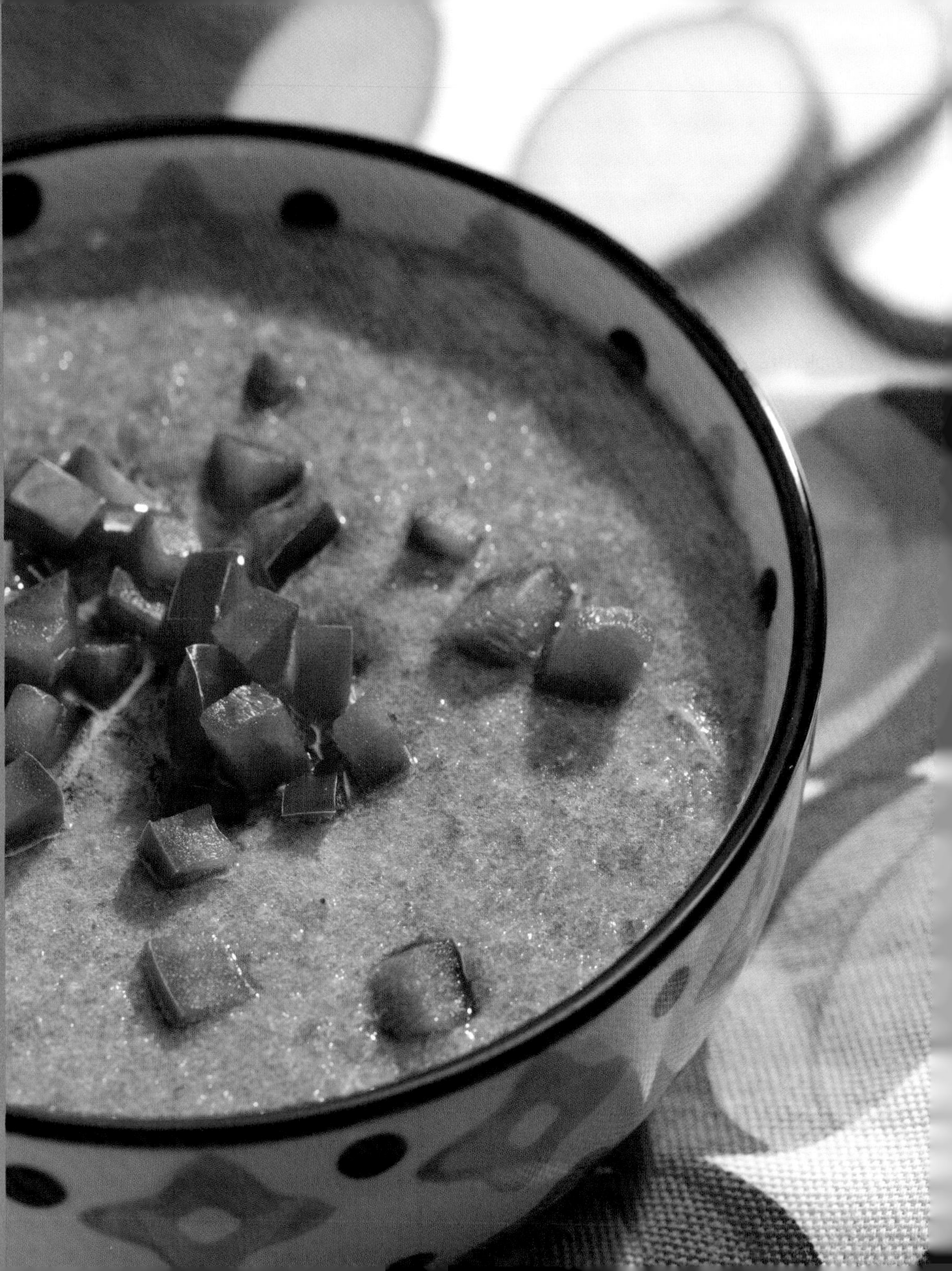

Cream of Greens Soup

A great way to enjoy your high-nutrient low-calorie green vegetables easily. Soup has been shown to support weight loss by helping to stimulate satiety hormones and reduce cravings. People have been shown to eat less when consuming foods in liquid form.

1 leek, sliced

2 cloves garlic, crushed

2 cups of vegetable stock

1 small head of broccoli, chopped

2 kale leaves, chopped

2 large handfuls of spinach leaves

1 zucchini, chopped

Handful of parsley

Salt and pepper (to taste)

Heat the oil on low heat; add leeks and garlic and slowly cook. Add the vegetable stock and vegetables (broccoli, kale, spinach, zucchini); slowly bring to a boil and cook until the zucchini is soft. The less you cook the vegetables, the better. Add salt and pepper to taste. Blend with a stick blender or blender and add the parsley. Garnish with chopped red pepper (optional).

2 servings | Amount Per Serving • % Daily Value

Serving Size 517g | Calories 131 | Calories from Fat 19 | Total Fat 2.1g • 3% | Trans Fat 0g | Cholesterol 0mg • 0% | Sodium 1417mg • 59% | Potassium 1051mg • 30% | Total Carbohydrates 20.3g • 7% | Dietary Fiber 5.1g • 21% | Sugars 5.8g | Protein 10.6g | Vitamin A 122% | Vitamin C 231% | Calcium 15% | Iron 20%

Rainbow
Salad

This salad features an array of nutrients due to the broad spectrum of deep-color produce that it contains. By consuming a rainbow of color, we are adding a high-nutrient profile to support good health.

Large handful of spinach
Large handful of beet leaves
1 small tomato, chopped
1 small cucumber, chopped
⅓ beet, grated
1 small carrot, grated
2 shallots, chopped
¼ red onion, sliced
¼ avocado, sliced
1 slice of pineapple or ½ an apple, chopped (optional)
2 tablespoons of hemp seeds (optional)

Mix and dress with ACV and Honey Vinaigrette dressing (below).

1 serving | Amount Per Serving • % Daily Value

Serving Size 680g | Calories 279 | Calories from Fat 95 | Total Fat 10.6g • 16% | Saturated Fat 2.2g • 11% | Trans Fat 0g | Cholesterol 0mg • 0% | Sodium 139mg • 6% | Potassium 1563mg • 45% | Total Carbohydrates 46.8g • 16% | Dietary Fiber 11.6g • 46% | Sugars 23.4g | Protein 6.4g | Vitamin A 279% | Vitamin C 79% | Calcium 14% | Iron 19%

Apple Cider Vinegar and
Honey Vinaigrette Dressing

Drizzle this zesty and sweet ACV vinaigrette over your favorite salads.

¼ cup of olive oil (extra virgin)

2 tablespoons of apple cider vinegar

1 tablespoon of water

1 teaspoon of honey

Salt and pepper (to taste)

Combine all ingredients and blend or mix well. The second portion can be stored for later use on Day 4.

2 servings | Amount Per Serving • % Daily Value

Serving Size 46g | Calories 230 | Calories from Fat 227 | Total Fat 25.2g • 39% | Saturated Fat 3.6g • 18% | Trans Fat 0g | Cholesterol 0mg • 0% | Sodium 292mg • 12% | Potassium 13mg • 0% | Total Carbohydrates 3.0g • 1% | Sugars 2.9g | Protein 0.0g | Vitamin A 0% | Vitamin C 0% | Calcium 0% | Iron 0%

Arugula and Fennel Salad

This is a light and green salad that has a delicious creamy dressing that is simple, tasty, and full of health-promoting nutrients. The salad dressing offers the healthy fats from the avocado with the health benefits of the ACV, which also adds an acidic element that compliments the meal.

1 large handful of baby kale leaves

1 large handful of arugula

½ fennel, finely sliced

½ cup cherry tomatoes, chopped in half

½ red bell pepper, chopped

⅛ red onion, thinly sliced

1 scallion, chopped roughly

4 strawberries, chopped (optional)

2 tablespoons of hemp seeds (optional)

Mix and dress with Goddess Dressing (below).

1 serving | Amount Per Serving • % Daily Value

Serving Size 298g | Calories 89 | Calories from Fat 6 | Total Fat 0.7g • 1% | Trans Fat 0g | Cholesterol 0mg • 0% | Sodium 39mg • 2% | Potassium 774mg • 22% | Total Carbohydrates 19.2g • 6% | Dietary Fiber 5.4g • 22% | Sugars 8.6g | Protein 3.7g | Vitamin A 164% | Vitamin C 275% | Calcium 11% | Iron 10%

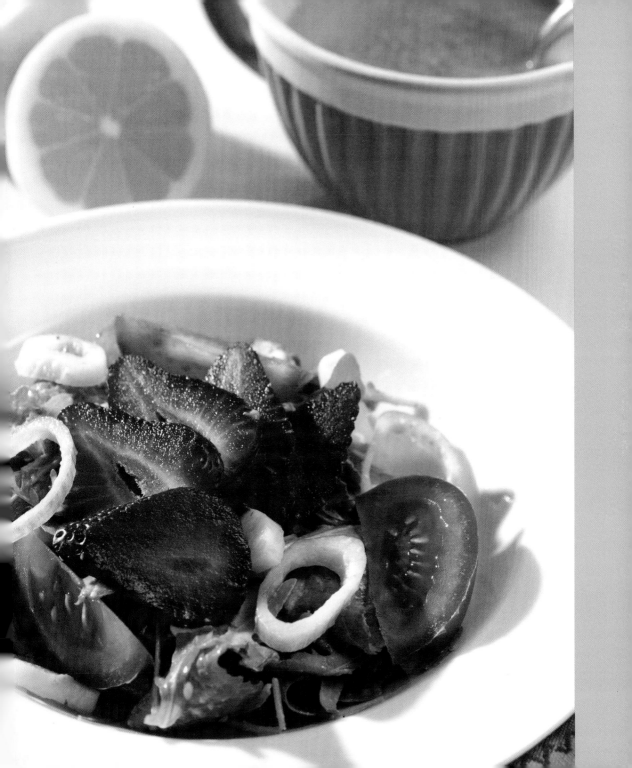

Goddess
Dressing

Lemony vinaigrette with smooth avocado, this Goddess Dressing goes perfectly on the Arugula and Fennel Salad.

½ **avocado, peeled and cored**

1 **tablespoon of apple cider vinegar**

1 **tablespoon of lemon juice**

¼ **teaspoon of salt**

¼ **cup of olive oil**

¼ **cup of water**

½ **teaspoon of dried oregano or basil (or 1 tablespoon fresh)**

3 **drops of stevia or ½ teaspoon honey (optional)**

Place all ingredients in a food processor and blend until smooth.

2 servings | Amount Per Serving • % Daily Value

Serving Size 95g | Calories 327 | Calories from Fat 316 | Total Fat 35.1g • 54% | Saturated Fat 5.7g • 29% | Trans Fat 0g | Cholesterol 0mg • 0% | Sodium 296mg • 12% | Potassium 260mg • 7% | Total Carbohydrates 6.0g • 2% | Dietary Fiber 3.4g • 14% | Sugars 1.9g | Protein 1.0g | Vitamin A 1% | Vitamin C 14% | Calcium 1% | Iron 2%

Caprese
Salad

This is an all-time favorite and popular salad that features basil, avocado, fresh tomatoes and the balsamic vinegar. The ingredients all complement each other, offering a simple, easy-to-make side dish for a hot meal or a side salad to pair with a juice.

1 tomato, sliced thickly

1 small cucumber, sliced

Handful of basil leaves

½ avocado, sliced

6 green olives

2 tablespoons of hemp seeds (optional)

Drizzle salad with balsamic vinegar and olive oil and season with salt and pepper to taste.

1 serving | Amount Per Serving • % Daily Value

Serving Size 274g | Calories 212 | Calories from Fat 168 | Total Fat 18.7g • 29% | Saturated Fat 3.4g • 17% | Trans Fat 0g | Cholesterol 0mg • 0% | Sodium 224mg • 9% | Potassium 555mg • 16% | Total Carbohydrates 12.5g • 4% | Dietary Fiber 5.1g • 21% | Sugars 3.6g | Protein 2.5g | Vitamin A 15% | Vitamin C 24% | Calcium 6% | Iron 10%

Note: Grapefruit may not be advised when taking some medications. It is always best to check with your doctor. You can substitute limes or lemons for the grapefruit. If any ingredient doesn't agree with you, then please use the substitution guide.

Do I have to follow the meal plan exactly?

No, but stick to the ACV guidelines described at the beginning of this book. For any meal, salad, smoothie, or juice, you can swap things around within one day or over the course of the week if you feel like eating something else on the menu. You may feel like eating a different snack or smoothie on the menu rather then what it says for that particular meal. That's okay.

Please feel free to adjust the plan to your liking with the guidelines in place to ensure you get the results you want and need. Using the substitution list can also be very helpful when you need to swap something with an alternative. This plan is not completely rigid but for this short period of time it needs to have strong guidelines to ensure you experience success. Replacing one plant-based meal with another is perfectly fine to do.

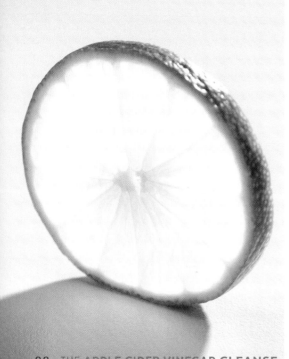

Alternative Recipes

These can be included as alternatives to similar recipes on the plan or if you prefer these as an alternative meal or snack. These can also be incorporated in the pre-Cleanse and post-Cleanse stages along with the recipes on the plan.

Tangy **Red**
Juice

This is an antioxidant rich juice that contains an array of nutrients. This juice is especially high in vitamin C, bioflavonoids, anthocyanins, carotenoids and other flavonoids. This is a great energy boosting juice while also refreshing and tasty.

2 oranges

2 carrots

2 celery sticks

1 beet

1 lemon

1 inch of fresh ginger

Wash all produce well. Peel the fruit and process all produce through the juicer. Enjoy!

1 serving | Amount Per Serving • % Daily Value (Juiced)

Serving Size 688g | Calories 158 | Calories from Fat 8.6 | Total Fat 1g • 2.7% | Saturated Fat 0.2g • 0.8% | Trans Fat 0g | Cholesterol 0mg | Sodium 199mg • 13.3% | Potassium 1319mg • 28.1% | Total Carbohydrate 49.4g • 38% | Dietary Fiber 1.8g • 4.7% | Sugars 31.4g | Protein 5.6g | Vitamin A 82% | Vitamin C 135.2% | Calcium 15.8% | Iron 23.9%

Apple Pie
Smoothie

The sweetness of the apples with added spices make this Apple Pie Smoothie taste just like homemade dessert. Cinnamon has amazing blood sugar-regulating benefits and can help to reduce cravings for sweet unhealthy foods. If you like apple pie, then you will enjoy this smoothie.

1 cup of coconut water
½ banana (fresh or frozen)
½ Granny Smith apple
1 handful of ice
1 tablespoon of chia seeds
¼ teaspoon of cinnamon
Pinch of nutmeg
Pinch of clove powder or 1 clove
1 teaspoon of honey or stevia (optional)

Wash, chop, and blend.

1 serving | Amount Per Serving • % Daily Value

Serving Size 265g | Calories 212 | Calories from Fat 26 | Total Fat 2.9g • 4% | Trans Fat 0g | Cholesterol 0mg • 0% | Sodium 27mg • 1% | Potassium 826mg • 24% | Total Carbohydrates 50.3g • 17% | Dietary Fiber 6.5g • 26% | Sugars 37.5g | Protein 2.4g | Vitamin A 1% | Vitamin C 161% | Calcium 13% | Iron 11%

Roasted
Cauliflower

I'm a big cauliflower fan due to its creamy taste. It's loaded with important cancer-fighting compounds and helps to support liver health. Roasting cauliflower gives it an enjoyable texture and changes the flavor completely. Adding additional spices can also make this a delicious side dish to enjoy!

½ head of cauliflower, chopped into large bite-size pieces
2 garlic cloves, crushed
2 teaspoons of coconut oil or olive oil
Season with salt and pepper (to taste)

Preheat oven to 400°F (200°C) and line a baking tray with parchment paper. Toss ingredients together and arrange on the baking tray. Cook for 25–30 minutes.

2 servings | Amount Per Serving • % Daily Value

Serving Size 74g | Calories 61 | Calories from Fat 43 | Total Fat 4.8g • 7% | Saturated Fat 0.7g • 3% | Cholesterol 0mg • 0% | Sodium 20mg • 1% | Potassium 213mg • 6% | Total Carbohydrates 4.5g • 2% | Dietary Fiber 1.7g • 7% | Sugars 1.6g | Protein 1.5g | Vitamin A 0% | Vitamin C 53% | Calcium 2% | Iron 2%

Baked
Mushrooms

Baked Mushrooms are a great pizza substitute! You can load the mushrooms up with delicious flavors without all the unnecessary starch and unhealthy fats that a normal pizza base can contain. Mushrooms offer a range of nutrients including B vitamins, potassium, selenium and vitamin D.

2 large Portobello mushrooms, stems removed and chopped

2 tablespoons of tomato paste

1 garlic clove, crushed

¼ teaspoon of oregano

1 tablespoon of fresh basil, chopped finely

2 scallions, chopped

1 tomato, chopped

6 kalamata olives, chopped

Salt and pepper (to taste)

Preheat oven to 400°F (200°C) and line a baking tray with parchment paper. In a large bowl, combine all of the ingredients, including the mushroom stems. Scoop the filling into the mushroom tops and drizzle them with olive oil. Bake in the oven for 20 minutes.

2 servings | Amount Per Serving • % Daily Value

Serving Size 176g | Calories 58 | Calories from Fat 14 | Total Fat 1.5g • 2% | Cholesterol 0mg • 0% | Sodium 119mg • 5% | Potassium 426mg • 12% | Total Carbohydrates 8.5g • 3% | Dietary Fiber 2.5g • 10% | Sugars 1.2g | Protein 4.1g | Vitamin A 11% | Vitamin C 15% | Calcium 3% | Iron 7%

Roasted **Beet**
Soup

This Roasted Beet Soup is a wholesome, warming meal. The added chili powder gives the sweetness of the beets an extra kick.

2 medium beets, trimmed

1 tablespoon of coconut oil

1 red onion, chopped

1 small sweet potato, chopped

2 garlic cloves, crushed

2 cups vegetable stock

Salt and pepper (to taste)

Pinch of chili powder

Preheat oven to 350°F (180°C). Wrap the beets in foil and bake for 50–60 minutes, or until tender. Once cooled, chop the beets. Heat oil in a saucepan over medium heat and sauté the onion, sweet potato, and garlic for 7 minutes. Add beets, vegetable stock, salt, pepper and chili powder. Cover and bring to a boil , and then simmer for 20 minutes. Transfer the soup to a blender and blend until it is smooth.

2 servings | Amount Per Serving • % Daily Value

Serving Size 463g | Calories 219 | Calories from Fat 77 | Total Fat 8.5g • 13% | Saturated Fat 6.3g • 31% | Cholesterol 0mg • 0% | Sodium 1445mg • 60% | Potassium 875mg • 25% | Total Carbohydrates 28.8g • 10% | Dietary Fiber 5.1g • 21% | Sugars 14.7g | Protein 8.5g

Substitutions

Substitutions may be needed due to allergies, dietary restrictions (such as medication use), time of year, costs of produce, personal preferences, and various other reasons.

Any green can be substituted for another green, while most fruits can be substituted for another similar fruit. It is best to use something that is similar in color and flavor.

Here is a basic substitution guide that matches the plan:

This:	For:
Apple	Pears, pineapple
Arugula	Watercress, spinach, kale, lettuce
Avocado	Choko, pineapple, banana, cucumber
Beet leaves	Romaine, spinach, kale
Beets (beetroot)	Red cabbage, carrot, golden beets
Bell pepper	Tomato, celery, carrot
Blueberries	Raspberries, cherries, blackberries
Broccoli	Kale, cauliflower, cabbage, Brussels sprouts
Carrot	Sweet potato, butternut squash, golden beets
Cauliflower	Broccoli, cabbage, Brussels sprouts
Chard	Spinach, kale, romaine, watercress
Cherries	Raspberries, blueberries, blackberries
Cucumber	Celery, celeriac root, zucchini
Fennel	Cucumber, celery, chicory
Grapefruit	Lemons, lime
Green beans	Zucchini
Kale	Spinach, chard, romaine
Leek	Scallions, white onion
Lemon	Lime, grapefruit
Lime	Lemon, grapefruit
Olives	Gherkins

This:	For:
Onions	Choose another variety—scallions, spring onions, chives
Orange	Mandarin, tangelos, ruby grapefruit
Pear	Apples, pineapple
Pineapple	Pear, apple, yellow grapefruit
Romaine	Kale, spinach
Spinach	Kale, chard
Strawberries	Raspberries, blueberries, blackberries
Tomato	Cherry tomatoes, red bell pepper, zucchini
Zucchini	Winter squash, eggplant, green beans

Special Note: The substitution may not always suit the recipe, so omit it completely and include more of all the other ingredients in a situation where substitutions are not suitable or available.

Optional plant protein additions

If you want to increase nutrients and protein, add in extra hemp seeds and/or spirulina. Spirulina is easy to consume in liquid, while seeds can be sprinkled on soups, on salads, in dressings, or in dips.

Strong flavors

If any of the juices have a flavor that is too strong for you, then you can add more of the ingredients that you do enjoy and less of the ones you don't, or simply substitute them. As you progress, your palate will change, and you will become more sensitive to sweetness. If you find beets too earthy, then thickly peeling them can help with the flavor. If any of the juices are too sour, then put a little more fruit in them or try watering them down. Adding ice to juices or smoothies can also reduce some of the stronger flavors.

chapter 4. Sticking to Your ACV Cleanse

Questions and Considerations for the 7-Day ACV Cleanse

What to do if you're still very hungry!

If you find that the plan leaves you still feeling famished, remember to eat more of the foods suggested, include another juice or vegetable snack, or add a soup or salad. Most of these meals are light. Be careful not to overeat very sweet fruits and avocados if you're looking to lose weight. Include these foods when instructed, but watch the quantity if weight loss is slow. Another tip is to drink more water and include strongly flavored herbal teas such as peppermint, spearmint, licorice, cinnamon, or ginger. You could even add an extra serving of ACV in water or club soda.

Another helpful option is to add extra bulking fibers to your water, juices, or smoothies. You can add things like chia seeds or psyllium husks (1 teaspoon). These slow digestion and give you a feeling of fullness.

Weather

I understand that if it is cold, you may not feel like eating salads, but I highly recommend it. Once you get used to it, it can be very enjoyable. Slightly cooking some of the ingredients can help with this, as can serving a warm salad containing things like roasted beets and carrots (rather than fresh varieties). Soups in summer may also not be too appetizing, so you can consume more salad options and enjoy the cooling gazpacho more often. I personally love salads and soups regardless of the weather.

Can I have dessert?

Yes, you can consume a piece of fruit or a small fruit salad, preferably berries/strawberries, chopped apple, or a juice. Herbal teas that are naturally sweetened (or slightly sweetened with stevia) are also okay.

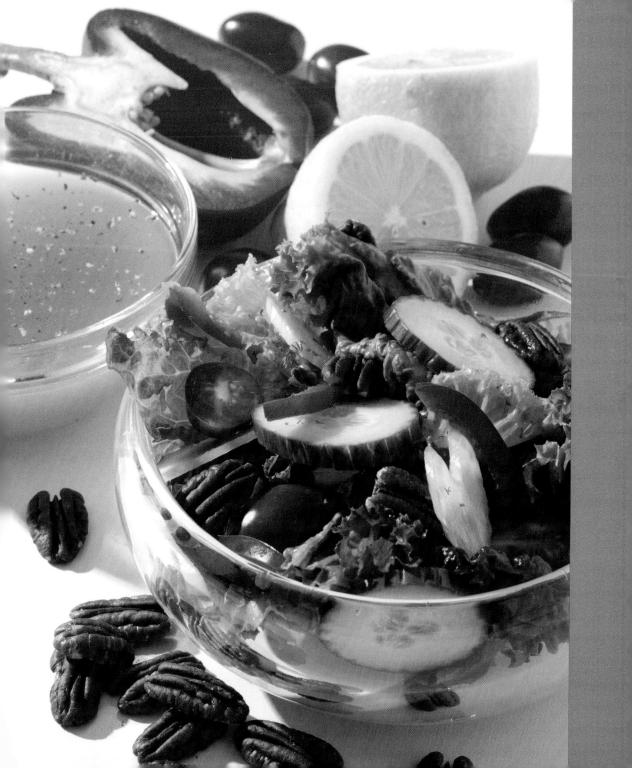

It's too much food for me

If you want to reduce the food intake, then just pick one option for each meal suggestion. If you're happy to consume less than instructed just make sure you have the juice suggestions. The juices are the top priority due to the health changes and support they give you.

If your weight isn't budging

Weight loss plateaus can happen at any point during a weight loss plan; they can, unfortunately, happen right at the beginning. It's more common for a plateau to hit after several weeks. Unfortunately, when the plateau hits, many people give up and convince themselves they have a slow metabolism or the new healthy eating plan doesn't work, and then they QUIT. People may feel frustrated if they feel they have been working hard and doing all the right things, and they are still not seeing the results they want. This is absolutely understandable!

As the body is readjusting to the diet and hormonal changes are occurring, this shift can stall an immediate change in your weight, but with persistence, your weight will start to fall again.

Here are some great tips to get it moving again:

- **Constipation**—The sudden increase of plant-based foods and fiber in the diet may trigger changes in regularity. As a result, constipation can slow down weight loss. See tips on how to treat constipation on page 110.

- **Exercise**—This certainly supports improved blood sugar and weight loss. Get moving, even if it's 3 times a week for 10 minutes or twice a week for 15 minutes. Just do something. Shake it up and try new exercises if you are already exercising so you won't get bored!

- **Hydration**—Water has a powerful effect on weight loss, so drink up!

- **Sleep**—Make sure you are getting your 7–9 hours of sleep every night to support weight loss.

- **Not enough food or JUICES**—Yes, that's right. Load on those low-calorie, high-nutrient foods to get the best effect to support a healthy metabolism.

- **Replacing whole food meals with extra juices**—This could budge any weight that isn't moving.

- **Add extra fiber**–Add 1 teaspoon of chia or psyllium husk to water, juice, or smoothies to increase a sense of fullness.

- **Stop stressing**–Stress makes our bodies store fat. If we are in a bad or stressful situation, our bodies think they need to store fat for an emergency. It's a very primitive reaction to stress, so let's get relaxed!

- **Think healthy**–If we change our perception of ourselves and see ourselves as a vital healthy human being, then we are very likely to get there.

And most of all, BE PATIENT!

Stay strong and motivated and know that even if the scale isn't moving as quickly as you want it to, your body is still achieving great things, which in the long run, means you'll have more sustainable weight loss and a healthier lifestyle.

It is important to understand that weight loss plateaus are a normal part of any long-term weight loss plan. I've seen them happen with clients for short periods of time and for others a little longer. Remember they are normal.

There are so many factors that contribute to weight loss plateaus:

- **Length of time the extra weight has been carried**

- **Age**–the older you are, the more difficult it can be

- **Sex**–men tend to lose weight faster due to hormones and muscle mass

- **Hormonal imbalances**–estrogen, cortisol, and insulin all play a role, along with other important hormones.

- **Thyroid disorders**–hypothyroidism causes weight gain

- **Insulin resistance and diabetes**–tendency to gain weight

- **Liver health**–fatty infiltration can slow it down

- **Cellular toxicity**–the more toxins there are in your body, the slower the weight loss will be

Despite all of these possible issues, it is absolutely necessary to maintain and support weight loss by keeping at it and never quitting on yourself or your health. What's going on inside is much more important than what is happening on the outside. Remember the outside follows the inside.

If visceral fat is a factor, as it often is in cases of fatty liver infiltration and pot-bellies, the body needs to burn the fat off in the visceral cavity as it does anywhere else in the body. This fat can't be seen without an ultrasound or an MRI, but as it reduces, so will the subcutaneous fat. This fat is not evident on the scales when it is being lost.

It's also important to note that as you lose weight, your results will naturally begin to slow down a little, as slimmer people tend to burn fewer calories.

Is it just all water weight that I've lost?

Has anyone noticed right at the beginning of a weight loss plan that the weight just drops off dramatically then stops or slows down after a day or so? You've probably heard from people that it's just water weight and not real weight loss, and they're kind of right, but fat loss is also occurring simultaneously.

It's important to understand that our body's water weight is regulated by many factors, which include hormones, hydration levels, sodium intake, electrolyte status, calorie intake, climate, physical activity, age, weight, sex, physical stress, and emotional stress.

During the initial stages of any good weight loss program, rapid weight loss is completely normal for many people. When your calories are reduced, your body gets its required energy by releasing and burning stores of glycogen, which is a type of stored sugar found in the muscles and the liver. Glycogen holds onto water, so when glycogen is burned up for energy, it also releases the water it contains. This contributes to the initial rapid weight loss that may accompany calorie reduction or macronutrient changes in the diet. During this initial weight loss, your body will also be burning up your fat stores as an energy source, and this will continue on as you continue your dietary changes. Once you're in for a few days and you're consistent, the rapid weight loss will slow down; this is when you start burning fat. This water weight loss doesn't necessarily occur for everyone, as varying factors affect it (as listed above).

Isn't fast weight loss bad?

How many times do we hear that it's better and safer to lose weight slowly? This, unfortunately, is an ideology and theory rather than a scientific fact. Studies indicate that it doesn't matter if the weight is lost slowly or quickly; what matters is what people do after they have lost the weight. Losing weight and then falling back into old unhealthy habits will cause rebound weight gain, whether you lost it quickly or slowly. One study that was published in the The Lancet Diabetes & Endocrinology in Australia showed that it didn't matter whether participants were placed on a rapid weight loss program or a gradual weight loss program for long-term weight control, although more than 80% of those in the rapid weight loss group achieved their target weight loss, versus just 50% in the gradual program.

Factors That Stimulate and Support a Healthy Metabolism

It's often believed that if someone is struggling with their weight, that they have a slow metabolism, but a slow metabolism is almost never the case. Dietary choices can have a supportive or destructive effect on your metabolism and the health of your hormones, liver, and digestive system, which all play a significant role in the way our bodies burn or store fat. The number of calories your body uses to carry out your normal, everyday processes is your basal metabolic rate.

Factors that affect your basal metabolic rate include your body size, muscle mass, sex, age, genetics, hormonal health, and some chronic health conditions, such as insulin resistance, fatty liver disease, and hypothyroidism.

There are many plant-based foods that we know support and stimulate the metabolism that I have included in the ACV cleanse along with the powerful properties of ACV.

Some metabolic foods to mention:

- **Chili**—The compound found in chili called capsaicin has a thermogenic effect; this means it causes the body to burn extra calories when eaten. Studies indicate that capsaicin may help fight obesity by decreasing caloric intake, shrinking fat tissue, and lowering fat levels in the blood.
- **Ginger**—In one study, when rats were fed ginger, they lost weight while consuming a high-fat diet.
- **Grapefruit**—Grapefruit contains many compounds that support and improve insulin sensitivity and help to maintain a healthy weight. A study showed that the consumption of fresh grapefruit juice caused a 3.5 lb weight reduction over 12 weeks, while the placebo group lost 0.6 lbs.

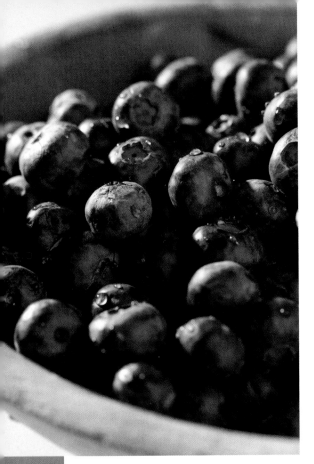

• **Lemons**—The polyphenols in lemons have been shown to improve serum insulin, glucose, and leptin levels significantly, thereby improving weight control. Lemons also support digestion and the production of bile.

• **Blueberries**—A study showed belly fat loss with the consumption of blueberries.

Herbal Tea to Support Your ACV Cleanse and Your Health:

Chamomile tea has a soothing effect on digestive irritation and is helpful for diarrhea, reflux, and abdominal cramps. It can also be helpful for nausea and can be consumed for painful periods (dysmenorrhea). It is also beneficial as a nerve relaxant.

Peppermint tea is particularly helpful for gas and flatulence, as it helps to relax the intestines, can assist with digestion, and has an intestinal soothing effect. It can also be very beneficial for reducing heartburn and morning sickness.

Fennel tea can particularly be beneficial for bloating and indigestion.

Dandelion root can be consumed as a roasted coffee substitute and has a beneficial effect on bile production and digestion; it can also be useful for constipation.

Licorice is not only useful for sugar cravings, but it also has a demulcent soothing effect in the digestive system. Licorice is used in herbal medicine as a healing tonic for gastrointestinal irritations and ulcerations.

Cinnamon is beneficial for blood sugar levels and has been well researched in the treatment of diabetes and insulin resistance; it also has some lovely warming aspects that aid digestion.

Ginger is great to add to hot water, morning tea, juices, smoothies, and meals. The list of healing properties is enormous! Ginger aids and supports digestion, nausea, arthritic pain and inflammation, poor circulation, blood sugar irregularities, painful periods, upper respiratory infections, lung disease, migraines, gut infections, and morning sickness. It has also been shown to be beneficial in liver disease.

Lemongrass is good for digestive complaints, such as bloating and flatulence. It is also helpful for headaches and nervous exhaustion.

Lemon Balm—I love this herb. Well, I love a lot of them, to be honest. This herb helps to reduce tension, nervousness, and mild cases of depression. Relax with a cup before bedtime to help you fall asleep.

Passionflower has gentle sedating qualities to help anxiety-related insomnia.

There are so many healing wonderful tea blends available, and I always encourage patients and people I know to include these for their refreshment and hydration as well as the natural health benefits that they provide.

It's important to find blends that are natural, preferably organic, and most importantly, ones that you enjoy drinking; with continued use comes the health-promoting benefits.

Food Addictions

The food industry has some serious science behind why "once you pop you can't stop." The food industry spends millions each year creating and formulating foods that stimulate a very short "bliss point" that doesn't last more than a few split seconds, so you have to keep eating to continue to get that bliss experience. This creates an urge to binge and causes people to overeat. These foods are also designed to let you think you haven't eaten very much, since they don't fill you up. Light, crunchy foods give you a false sense of not having eaten much; it's a perfect combination to make you eat more than you need, thus increasing the sales of junk food.

It's all a chemical trick that affects our satiety and appetite centers in the brain in a way that natural food does not do. Food that is dense in calories fills you up for long periods and creates true satisfaction and appetite control.

Consuming healthy foods and resetting your system with ACV will help you eliminate unhealthy processed foods from your diet. For some people, the only way to truly heal and reverse diseases is to stop eating these foods entirely to allow your body to heal. Eventually, this will help you stop having cravings and will repair the relationship between your body and food.

The Importance of Emotional Health

This may feel like a period of deprivation, but it is beneficial to have a positive mindset about what a wonderful opportunity this is to gain better health, improve your nutritional knowledge, and lose weight. Concentrating on the positive things about the 7-Day ACV Cleanse will help you to be more successful.

Make a point of appreciating and enjoying what you are consuming with your palate, your eyes, and your mind. I love to observe the bright colors that nutritionally dense food has to offer. The bright color is nature's way of telling us that the food is jam-packed with energizing nutrients and phytocompounds that have a myriad of health benefits.

Beautifully colored food offers an array of specialized compounds that offer the longest list of health benefits. Think turmeric for its anti-inflammatory benefits, with its strong yellow pigments, or blueberries, which are known to prevent cognitive decline and to have anti-aging benefits, and beets for their exercise performance-enhancing qualities and liver detoxification benefits.

Make a point of understanding where true hunger ends and emotional hunger begins. Remember that emotional hunger is sudden, food specific, and won't be quelled with a normal-sized healthy meal, while physical hunger is gradual, will be satisfied with most things, and there is no urgency. Emotional hunger comes with frustration, boredom, stress, and loneliness and can also come with a sense of self-reward.

Emotional connections to food and eating for comfort are considered normal and common. But if you give in to these cravings frequently, it can be problematic. Being able to recognize when it's happening is the first step forward in breaking the habit. Finding alternative activities that are comforting and supportive for yourself is another step forward.

As a practitioner, I believe it's important to cover the reasons why people overeat and why they may gravitate toward the worst food offenders. Talking to loved ones or trusted professionals and creating an environment that is supportive to you are paramount in your success.

Detox Symptoms from the ACV Cleanse

It certainly seems odd: we get healthy, change our diets, increase our fruit and vegetable consumption, reduce our sugar, stop drinking alcohol, and start exercising and we feel worse! We might feel confused or weak. This is not unusual. Detox symptoms, as they are commonly known, can occur for varying reasons. Any type of healthy dietary change can cause some "detox" symptoms. Some of these changes include:

- Calorie reduction
- Withdrawal from caffeine, sugar, processed foods, alcohol and food additives
- The breakdown of fat-soluble chemicals, aka "toxins," which are stored in fatty tissue. This includes organs like the liver; side effects occur as the "toxins" recirculate back into the bloodstream and are broken down by the normal liver processes and are removed via the kidney, skin, and bowel.
- Stimulating liver function and increasing bile flow may also cause some nausea, indigestion, and general discomfort

Some pre-existing health issues can become aggravated in the early stages of the ACV Cleanse. Health problems can often become worse before they get better. This is commonly known as a "healing crisis." This can be more evident for skin problems where breakouts or rashes may become aggravated. Fatigue can also be exacerbated and digestive symptoms can worsen. If you are armed with the right tools, you can combat these symptoms. My weakness is my skin; it has a little breakout every time I do a cleanse, but it comes back better than ever after those first few days.

How long can cleansing symptoms last?

1–3 days is the normal amount of time that these symptoms can last, while some people may experience none at all, particularly those that have prepared adequately or who have always maintained a very healthy diet. Others may have them for a longer period of time. It is also important to know that if anything concerns you or seems unusual at any point, then it is best to see your doctor or health care professional.

Lack of preparation—The more processed foods and high-sugar foods you consume prior to the 7-Day ACV Cleanse, the more symptoms you may experience. After some time consuming the right foods that support good health, you will begin to feel better.

Calorie restriction—If you reduce your calories, the body will have something to say about it! The bodily complaints may be uncomfortable at first, but it is easy to get on top of them with high-fiber nutrient-dense foods, rest, fluids, and ACV.

Your diet was high in processed chemical-laden foods—As your body detoxes away from highly refined foods, MSG, and other addictive additives, your energy, cravings, and mood levels may be affected initially.

Caffeine withdrawal—Caffeine is a highly addictive substance and removing it, or even cutting it down, may cause symptoms like headaches, fatigue, and moodiness.

Sugar withdrawal—If you consume processed sugar regularly, you are more likely to experience side effects. Sugar withdrawals can include headaches, lethargy, muscle aches and pains, irregular blood sugar levels, moodiness, irritability, sleep disturbances, dizziness, and more. Sugar is certainly one of the most addictive foods you can consume and has been compared to many drugs due to its highly addictive qualities.

On a positive note, once you are off sugar, your cravings and your taste for processed sugar will become less and less prevalent. Nutrients, ACV, and the plan will support improved blood sugar levels, improved mood, and improved digestion, and reduced cravings. Sugar is a monster that you can never master; the more sugar you eat, the more sugar you want, so let's get off it for good!

Blood sugar irregularities—These also apply to people who experience hypoglycemia, insulin resistance, diabetes, and those who eat too many carbohydrates to support their erratic blood sugar levels. As your body starts to burn fat, your hormones will readjust. With the consumption of more fruits and vegetables, ACV, and healthy whole foods, your blood sugars should stabilize.

Heredity—Genetic predisposition to certain health complaints, such as headaches, skin conditions, sinusitis, and digestive complaints, can make you experience symptoms in the initial stages of the ACV Cleanse.

Fatty liver or inflamed liver—If you have an underfunctioning or sluggish liver due to fatty infiltration or gallbladder disturbances, then a cleanse program may initially cause some symptoms. Follow the guidelines to support your health and body as much as possible.

I certainly don't want to tell you about possible symptoms to be all doom and gloom, but with years of experience supporting people through programs, I know that if you are armed with the information about what symptoms you can potentially expect, then you are more likely to be successful. The time when most people give up is during the first few days, when they might experience symptoms. But the solution might be as simple as a cup of water or an extra serving of fruit or vegetables. Often, the best solution is the simplest solution. I certainly do not advocate that anyone push on if they feel very unwell, are very uncomfortable, or feel concerned. Always remember to consult your doctor or health care professional if you have concerns.

What symptoms can occur?

Feeling cold—This is due to calorie restriction (in my experience this also normally means weight loss is happening); drink warming beverages with optional spices, take a warming bath, and wear extra clothing.

Dizziness—This can be due to hydration levels, blood pressure changes, and blood sugar irregularities.

Cravings—As you stop ingesting specific foods and reduce your calories, you may experience cravings for all sorts of unusual things. I remember my first experience was a craving for a donut that lasted an hour! I haven't really eaten many in my life (maybe as a teenager I had a few), and I actually don't like them, as I have associations of flour in hot rancid cooking oil (not appetizing to me at all). The point is that my unconscious mind picked up something that was highly refined and had a high glycemic index that could re-establish its glycogen stores ASAP. This is the absolute worst solution, but it's important to know that it will pass and is less likely to occur if you eat according to the plan. I'd gotten too busy and had fallen behind in the plan. This is why I'm so strict with time frames and consuming what's listed.

Headaches—These are almost always caused by dehydration, even if you feel that you have consumed enough healthy fluids. Keep drinking water and adding extra electrolytes, which will normally eliminate or reduce the headache. A reduction in sodium can also alter your electrolyte balance.

Blood sugar irregularities—Hypoglycemia, insulin resistance, and diabetic conditions all indicate impaired glucose metabolism. If you are diabetic, it is important to always check your blood sugar and always talk to your doctor about any changes that you make. Eating small, frequent meals and staying hydrated are important. You can add extra plant-based snacks to the plan if required. Adding in extra plant-based protein, such as hemp protein powder or seeds, spirulina, or a vegan protein powder, can also help.

Increased urination—If you normally don't drink a lot of healthy fluids and water, then when you start this plan you may feel that you are running off to the toilet way too often. Don't fret; this will pass as your bladder adjusts to the increased fluid intake. Another reason that this happens is that you are shedding water weight. This is normal; as glycogen stores are depleted, water goes with them.

Digestive upsets—Bloating, indigestion, diarrhea, constipation, and flatulence may occur when on the ACV Cleanse, as any dietary change can cause a disturbance in your normal bowel and stomach patterns. For solutions, see below.

Skin breakouts and rashes—Since the skin is the largest eliminative organ, when we make big changes to our diet, our skin may initially suffer as our bodies start to regulate our detoxification pathways, which of course include the skin. Sweat it out and drink more water. Making a mask and using your ACV as a toner will certainly help to reduce this effect.

Fatigue—This can be due to a reduction in calories, lack of hydration, irregular blood sugar, or withdrawal from certain substances, such as refined carbohydrates, caffeine, or sugar. Once your body has adjusted to these changes, your energy levels will soar.

Aches and pains—These are common! Causes include calorie restriction, electrolyte disturbances, dehydration, and/or blood sugar changes.

Brain fatigue or brain fog—This is commonly caused by a reduction in calories, sugar, and/or caffeine. It is important to keep hydrated.

White coating on tongue or in mouth—This can be due to gut flora irregularities and dietary changes. Remember to clean not only your teeth but also your tongue. Take a probiotic. Using ACV as a mouthwash will certainly help to reduce this effect.

Solutions That Work and Troubleshooting Tips!

Drink more water—You may need to drink more than the common recommendation of 8 cups. Keep an eye on your urine color and ensure it is a light straw color.

Up your electrolytes—This can be done with an extra serving of vegetable broth, coconut water, maple water, or a red or orange juice (make it 80% vegetables).

Include herbal teas—See more on teas for ailments in the Teas section.

Consume a vegetable or fruit snack—Eat a serving of cucumber, celery sticks, carrots, apple, pear, or pineapple.

Sit down and take a few deep, slow breaths.

Go for a walk outside—If it's possible, get outside for exercise, fresh air, and a new perspective.

Work on ways to deal with emotional upsets— Breathing exercises, talking to someone trusted, going to bed early, reading a great book, spending time on a favorite hobby, or doing another non-food-related activity can be a great way to take care of yourself emotionally. Emotional health can play a big part in how we take care of our physical well-being. I normally suggest creating a list of things that you know make you happy and keep this somewhere that you can look at daily. Make sure you are doing these things for yourself on a regular basis.

Peppermint oil—I wouldn't have believed it was so effective for a headache many years ago if it wasn't for someone dabbing it on my temples. Dabbing peppermint oil on your temples, the base of your skull, and over the area that is most afflicted will help reduce the pain. Dilute peppermint oil in an oil base like coconut oil if you have sensitive skin.

More on Digestive Upsets and Solutions

Digestive upsets can come from making any dietary change, such as including more fruits and vegetables in the diet, altering your fiber intake, or adding any new food to your diet.

It's important to note that preparation is likely to minimize these issues or prevent them from happening at all. These changes and aggravations are temporary, and with a few tips, we can avoid them.

DIARRHEA

You can prevent diarrhea by taking a broad-spectrum probiotic. A special beneficial yeast called *Saccharomyces boulardii* can be your best defense against diarrhea. It can be found in most good health food stores where probiotics and vitamins are found. It is a shelf-stable product; follow the instructions for the treatment of diarrhea. There are studies on how safe and effective it is in acute diarrhea for adults and children. Consuming green bananas can help reduce excessive motions due to the high starch content.

While diarrhea is occurring and shortly after it is over, it's important to re-establish your electrolytes and drink a sodium-based vegetable broth and/or coconut water along with extra fluids, such as ginger tea, chamomile tea, and filtered water.

Note: If any problems persist, it's important to talk to your doctor or health care professional.

CONSTIPATION

This is often listed as one of the most common health complaints; it is estimated that over 60 million people are affected in the U.S.

If you experience the following symptoms, you may be suffering from constipation: passing hard, dry stool, infrequent bowel movements, minor anal tears, the sensation that you have to "go" but nothing will come out, or feeling that you haven't emptied adequately. Other symptoms may include bloating, abdominal discomfort, pain, anal fissures, and hemorrhoids.

The most common causes of constipation include a lack of fiber, dehydration, a change in routine, lack of exercise, and repeatedly ignoring the urge to go. Other less obvious constipation causes are low thyroid function, magnesium deficiency, digestive infections, reduced healthy gut microbiota, stress, pregnancy, some medications (such a painkillers), IBS, food intolerances, and other more serious concerns, such as tumors.

Ideally, you should have a bowel motion daily to ensure a healthy colon and digestive system; regular motions are imperative to support a happy mood! The gut is often described as the second brain, as it supports the production of neurotransmitters, such as serotonin, one of our feel-good hormones.

Constipation may be an ongoing issue, or it may develop during the ACV Cleanse. Constipation may slow down weight loss and have a myriad of health associations, such as feeling lethargic, having a poor mood, or experiencing muscle aches and pains or headaches.

To treat constipation, do the following:

- Drink more water! It is important to help increase the fluid in the stool; this helps to bulk out the stool and softens it, so it is easier to pass. Keep in mind that the body will deliver fluid needs to the tissues and cells before it goes to the bowel.

- Add an extra serving of warm water, ACV, and lemon in the morning upon rising.

- Exercise regularly. Physical movement supports peristalsis (intestinal contractions) that move the stool through the colon.

- Take a broad-spectrum probiotic (this has a normalizing effect on bowel activity).

- Take a fiber supplement, such as psyllium husk, chia seeds, or flaxseeds. Take 1 tablespoon daily with at least 1–2 glasses of water. Consuming fiber without water can further aggravate constipation.

- Consume more magnesium-rich vegetables—such as kale, chard (silverbeet), spinach, and beet greens.

- Up the amount of fruits and vegetables that you consume.—This will give you more fiber and nutrients!

- Eat fermented foods or beverages, such as kefir, kombucha, sauerkraut, or kimchi.

- Eat extra beets in the juices and diet. Beets stimulate bile production, which in turn stimulates bowel movements.

- Make time for relaxation. Feeling tense can cause tension in the bowel, thus causing it to constrict; more stress equals less blood and nutrients that are being delivered to the bowel, thus slowing it down.

- Give yourself an abdominal massage in the direction of your bowel, which runs in a clockwise direction. A massage with oil can move things along due to gentle stimulation and movement.

Since food intolerances can also be a factor, keep this in mind when re-introducing foods back into the diet post-Cleanse.

DISCOMFORT OR NAUSEA

If a particular juice recipe or meal is obviously upsetting you, then it's best to dilute the juice down with water and/or coconut water and drink it in separate doses. Some juices can be very strong for a beginner, and everyone responds a little differently. Watering them down almost always reduces this effect.

Drinking smaller amounts more frequently throughout the day can be helpful.

Some ingredients may also be upsetting to you, so avoid any suspect ingredients and replace them with something more suitable.

Adding lemon and ginger to warm or hot water throughout the day can reduce nausea or any type of digestive cramping.

Consume calming herbal teas:

- **Fennel:** for bloating, indigestion

- **Chamomile:** for pain, discomfort, and indigestion

- **Peppermint/Spearmint:** for bloating, flatulence, IBS

- **Aniseed/Licorice:** for discomfort, bloating, and blood sugar irregularities

- **Marshmallow root tea:** for pain, discomfort, IBS. Dried roots need to simmer in a pot of water on the stovetop for 20 minutes and then the water needs to be strained before you consume it. This is a lovely, demulcent, healing, soothing tea.

- **Ginger**—for nausea, irritation, and digestive upsets

FLATULENCE

This can occur due to fiber changes and new vegetable and fruit additions.

Removing or reducing the gas-causing vegetables (cabbage, cauliflower, kale, Brussels sprouts, broccoli, onions, and garlic) can help reduce flatulence. This is due to the high sulfuric content of these vegetables.

It is important to note that cabbage juice has been traditionally used to heal and soothe ulcers and irritation, due to its glutamine content. In some cases, cabbage juice may help, rather than aggravate, your colon, but this will vary from person to person.

REFLUX

Avoid lying down directly after you have consumed any juices or meals. Ease off the spicy additions in any recipe or juice. Drink more water and consume herbal teas, such as fennel and chamomile. Consume less, more frequently, and get moving. Be cautious with acidic ingredients such as citrus, tomatoes, onions, and garlic.

How to Commit to the 7-Day Cleanse WITHOUT Losing Weight

This can be very important for people who want to improve their health or address a health condition but who don't want, or need, to lose weight.

You will have to add more food to the plan or add in more starchy plants and healthy fats.

Add in extra servings of:

- Baked starchy vegetables, including potatoes, sweet potatoes, pumpkins, turnips, parsnips, carrots, squash, and corn.
- Healthy fats, such as coconut oil, avocado, olive oil, and flaxseed oil.
- Smoothies that include coconut water, bananas, mangos, whole avocados, coconut oil, and/or other healthy oils.

Eat more frequently, and add in more juices along with the extra servings of foods until you find that spot where you are not losing weight.

The Importance of Hydration

Proper hydration supports:

- Energy production
- Exercise performance
- Weight loss
- Digestion
- Muscle health
- Brain function
- Reduced headaches
- Detoxification and bowel health
- Appetite regulation

Water is essential to all life on the planet; it's vital for nearly every metabolic function in the human body. The average human is approximately 65% water.

We lose fluid continuously throughout the day from skin evaporation, breathing, urine, and stool output. When your water intake is less than what you are losing, then you can become dehydrated. Dehydration can cause fatigue, poor concentration, hunger, lack of motivation, headaches, mood changes, dry lips and mouth, darkly colored urine, and in more serious cases, confusion, weakness, and hallucinations.

I highly recommend consuming adequate fluids during, before, and after the 7-Day Cleanse to ensure results and to reduce the occurrence of detox symptoms. When you are ingesting so many nutrients, your pathways of detoxification are regulated, allowing for the increased excretion of metabolic waste. We need that extra fluid to assist in the excretion processes through sweat, stool, and urine. Drinking enough water supports our natural ability to detoxify.

It is also very important to understand that you can overhydrate yourself (causing hyponatremia). Overhydration can cause a depletion of electrolytes in the body, which can have serious side effects, but it is a rare occurrence.

The ideal color of your urine to establish your level of hydration is a clear to very light straw color; this shows the dilution of your urinary waste metabolites.

HOW WATER HELPS WEIGHT LOSS

Water can increase satiety and boost your metabolic rate. A study that was performed at the Humboldt-University in Berlin, Germany showed that drinking around 2 cups (16 oz.) can increase metabolism by 24% for up to 1.5 hours. This equals an extra 100 calories per day that can be burned just by making sure you're drinking enough water.

The timing is important too, and drinking water half an hour before meals is the most effective. It can support feelings of fullness so that you eat fewer calories. In a small study at the Department of Human Nutrition, Foods, and Exercise, in Blacksburg, Virginia, it was found that people who drank 2 cups (16 oz.) of water before meals lost 44% more weight over a period of 12 weeks.

JAZZ UP YOUR WATER WITH THESE FLAT BELLY TIPS!

If you're not a water lover, and many aren't, mixing up your water flavors is a fun and healthy way to encourage the consumption of extra healthy fluids.

In a water jug (about 4–8 cups) add in any of the following ingredients and allow to steep for a few hours or overnight. Stirring occasionally can assist in the flavor enhancement.

- **Minty Berry Water**—a handful of mint leaves and ¼ cup of berries, chopped and steeped
- **Cucumber Water**—1 teaspoon of freshly grated ginger, 1 cucumber (sliced), ½ fresh lemon, and mint leaves
- **Strawberry Water**—strawberries (¼ cup) and ice
- **Sangria Water**—1 sliced apple, 1 sliced orange, ½ fresh lemon, ¼ cup of ACV (optional), and 1 teaspoon of honey (optional)
- **Sparkling Ginger Water**—Sparkling water, 1 teaspoon of grated ginger (optional), and a pinch of natural stevia or 1 teaspoon of honey
- **Sparkling Citrus Water**—sparkling water with ½ fresh lemon and/or ½ fresh lime

It can be fun to start thinking outside the box and jazz up your plain water with some fun and tasty ideas!

Feel free to experience with fruit- and vegetable-flavored water!

chapter 5. Life Post-Cleanse

How to Transition Back into a Healthy Eating Plan Post-Cleanse

It is important to slowly transition back into eating a healthy diet. During the pre-Cleanse period and the actual 7-Day ACV Cleanse, your appetite will have regulated back to a more consistent level with reduced cravings. When you reduce your calories below your body's requirements, the body burns fat. When this happens, the appetite and blood sugar levels tend to regulate more efficiently. This is when weight loss occurs.

When you have been following a healthy cleanse program, it is advisable to not just dive back into eating what you were eating previously, particularly if it contains too many of the not so healthy foods discussed in this book. If you go back to your old eating habits, this will cause rapid weight gain. It is advisable to slowly reintroduce the other food groups as suggested and to not overdo it post-Cleanse. It can be easy to undo all your benefits in a relatively short period of time if you jump back into eating certain foods in higher quantities.

You will also find that you will need less food to fill you up since you've changed your eating habits and cut your overall calorie consumption down during the cleanse.

Avoiding refined foods, sugars, and other unhealthy foods will reduce your appetite and improve your blood sugar levels along with the health benefits of the apple cider vinegar. Unfortunately, sugar and refined foods stimulate the appetite and create bigger cravings for more unhealthy foods. Remember to take your time re-introducing foods and continue eating a wide variety of plant-based nutrients and foods. To continue to reap the health benefits of the Cleanse over the long-term, consume 1 tablespoon of ACV three times daily before mealtime or include it in your recipes.

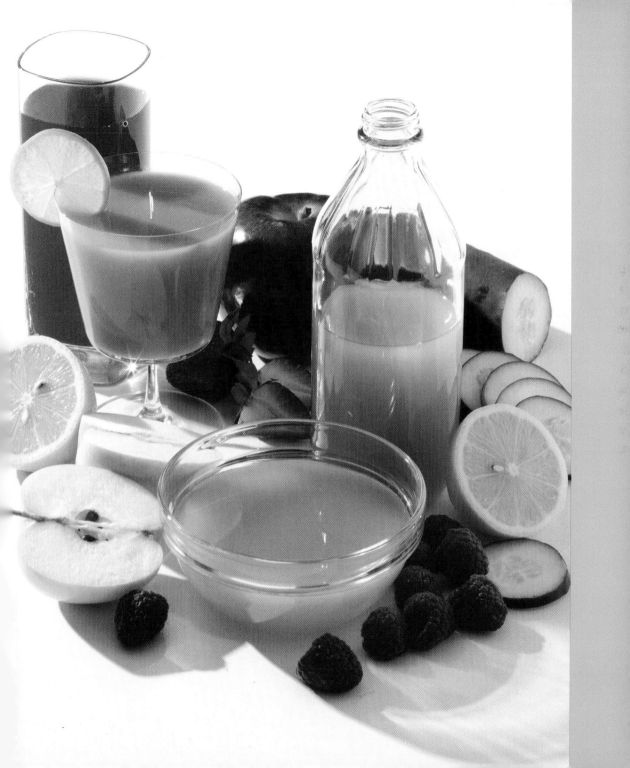

Guidelines for the Post-Cleanse Period

Days 1–2

Consume plenty of juices, smoothies, soups, and salads. You can increase your whole food consumption with extra soups, salads, fruits, vegetable-based meals, nuts, seeds, and gluten-free grains (quinoa, wild or brown rice, buckwheat and teff).

Days 3–5

Re-introduce protein sources, such as wild fish, organic eggs and poultry, and vegetarian sources of protein, such as beans, lentils, split peas, and tempeh.

Days 6–7

Re-introduce 100% grass-fed red meat and organic dairy if you choose to, along with gluten-containing grains (if tolerated).

If you want to challenge any possible food allergy or intolerance, then wait 2–4 more weeks before re-introduction. Continue to avoid the suspected food for a total of 4 weeks, and then re-introduce it with a challenge that includes 2–3 servings of the suspected food per day for 3 days to truly determine if the food is a problem. Keeping a diary helps to pinpoint any potential problems. Keep a record of bowel habits, energy levels, lethargy, digestive upset, nausea, indigestion, aches and pains, joint pain or inflammation, headaches, skin rashes, breathing complaints, or upper respiratory aggravation, such as nasal congestion, sinusitis, or rhinitis. Observe if there is any pattern.

Healthy Eating Over the Long Term

What a healthy day may look like

Breakfast—Fruit with organic yogurt and/or seeds and nuts, eggs with vegetables, a bowl of vegetables, salad, juice, soup, smoothie, oats or buckwheat porridge with fruit.

Morning snack—Juice, smoothie, vegetable snack, fruit, nuts, and seeds

Lunch—Vegetable dish with protein, salad with protein, smoothie, juice, soup (lunch must be vegetable based)

Afternoon Snack—Juice, smoothie, vegetable snack, fruit, nuts and seeds

Dinner—Protein source with loads of vegetables (like a salad or vegetable-based dish). Make sure 75% of your plate is covered in colorful vegetables!

Supper—Herbal tea

Remember to include ACV with each meal and enjoy a morning drink upon rising!

Additional Guidelines

You can commit to doing the ACV plan for another week if you would like to continue your ACV Cleanse results. You can also implement a pattern where you follow the plan for 2–3 days per week or fortnight to continue achieving results post-Cleanse.

You can do the 7-Day ACV Cleanse every 6–8 weeks on a long-term basis. The Cleanse is not a plan that you would follow continuously, as it's designed to be done on a short-term basis with healthier long-term eating and lifestyle guidelines to be followed as suggested.

It's All About Habits

A habit is something that you do automatically that takes very little thought or effort. It's easy and normal, and it's all on autopilot. Want to make something good a habit? Do it every day, at roughly the same time every day, and it will slowly become your new norm. If you forget or miss a few days, then just get right back into it and keep going. Often, people do something for a few days or a few weeks, but if you persist for a few months, then it will likely become a habit.

Healthy eating and healthy habits are made one day at a time, and sometimes one habit at a time! Just keep doing the same thing every day. If you need a reminder, you can set an alarm on your phone or make a list of daily habits that you keep somewhere highly visible in your home.

7 Suggested Healthy Daily Habits

These can be placed as reminders and alarms in your smart phone or listed somewhere that is highly visible to you!

On Rising—Drink 2 cups (16 oz.) of warm water with 1 fresh lemon and ACV.

Mid-Morning—Have a piece of fruit and drink 2 cups (16 oz.) of water.

Lunch—Eat a salad, plate of vegetables, or a juice.

Afternoon—Drink a juice.

Later Afternoon—Drink 2 cups (16 oz.) of water.

Daily—Include ACV with each meal.

Special daily reminder—Remind yourself how amazing you are and what a great job you are doing! You can do anything you want to do! If it's difficult for you to say that to yourself, then it's even more important to do it.

People don't get motivated with negative and demeaning self-talk; people succeed with supportive, positive thoughts and feelings. Positivity breeds more positivity.

Remember, if you want to be successful in changing your ways, think of your new habits as non-negotiable. Would you ever not brush your teeth or take your shower? Make these habits into must-dos no matter how busy you are, even if it's just one new thing!

There's an expression that says, "If you don't make time for health you will be making time for illness." This is so true! Take control of your health and always make time for your own wellness.

Exercising also falls into this category; the more you keep doing it regularly, the more your body will get used to the movement. Eventually, it will crave exercise.

Top 10 tips for healthy eating and weight control

- Drink 8 cups (2 liters) of water or more daily.
- Eat fiber-rich foods regularly to keep you feeling fuller for longer.
- Eat 8–13 servings of fruits and vegetables per day. I push for the upper limit.
- Consume 2–4 servings of fruit per day, depending on your calorie needs, with the rest being vegetables. Your diet should be 80% vegetables and 20% fruit.
- Consume a rainbow every day to ensure nutrient diversity and good health.
- Avoid all processed foods as much as possible; less is always better.
- Consume adequate protein and healthy fats every day.
- Get active to maintain a healthy lifestyle.
- Take time to relax and be happy.
- Get adequate rest every night.

The USDA's Dietary Guidelines recommend adults eat anywhere from 5 to 13 servings of fruits and vegetables per day. Make sure you eat at least 2 meals per day that include 50–75% colored vegetables and a fist-sized portion of protein from things like vegetarian proteins, eggs, poultry, or fish. For other meats, eat a palm-sized portion. See the protein section for ideas and amounts. The United States Department of Agriculture (USDA) sets the serving sizes for most fruits and vegetables at one cup.

Here are some examples of approximately 1 serving size:

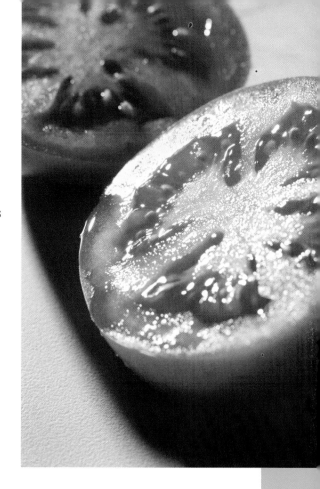

- 1 banana
- 8 large strawberries
- 2 large plums or apricots
- 1 medium apple
- 3 large broccoli spears
- 1 large carrot
- 1 large tomato
- 1 Lebanese cucumber
- ½ sweet potato
- 2 celery sticks
- 1 cup of raw greens and ½ cup of cooked greens such as spinach leaves
- 1 small pepper

Top 25 Tricks for Improved Weight Loss

Never get too hungry—Excess hunger encourages poor choices.

Snack smart—Eat vegetables and vegetable-based juices, nuts, fruit, and other healthy whole foods.

Spice it up–Chili, cinnamon, ginger, and turmeric have been shown to increase and support metabolic health.

Avoid artificial sweeteners–These increase cravings and have been shown to increase weight over the long-term.

Make it nutrient dense–Nutrient-dense foods are more satisfying.

Keep a diet diary–Being aware of what you are doing and monitoring your own patterns can be truly eye opening.

Eat slowly–Eating too quickly increases the likelihood that you will overeat.

Breathe out your cravings–A few deep breaths and waiting a few moments can reduce the urge to cave in to cravings.

Snooze to lose–The University of Pennsylvania found that even just a few nights of sleep deprivation can lead to almost immediate weight gain.

Plan ahead–You're less likely to make a poor decision if know what your next healthy meal or snack will be.

Stay well hydrated–Hydration helps maintain your metabolism and supports satiety.

Use smaller plates and utensils–Our plates have become larger than ever before, which means we fill them up. Use smaller plates to eat less.

Enjoy herbal teas–Teas that support blood sugar and metabolic health, such as green tea, matcha, licorice, spearmint, or cinnamon, can be an excellent evening treat.

Exercise–Make time for both resistance training and cardio exercises. Muscle burns at least four times as many calories as fat does; twenty minutes of strength training 2–3 times each week is enough to get positive results.

Liquid-based meals–Liquid meals like juices, smoothies, or soups can really help to cut back on the calories and fill you up fast.

Healthy starter–Consuming soup or a salad before a meal has been shown to cut overall calorie consumption. Foods with a liquid base or high vegetable base are correlated with improved satiety and decreasing your overall food intake at the next meal.

Avoid processed sugar—Any sugar-based snack or meal will only drive up your appetite and cravings and stimulate your fat-making hormones while inhibiting your fat-burning hormones.

Reward yourself—Reward yourself with something other than food. This is likely to create long-term healthy eating habits where food is enjoyable, but it's not used as an emotional reward. Reducing any unhealthy emotional relationships to food is always a very positive step forward.

Know your triggers—If ice cream is your weakness, then remove it from your home. If 3:00 p.m. hits and you run to the vending machine, then consume a healthy snack at 2:30 p.m. that fills you up. If you graze before dinner, then snack only on vegetable sticks. Create a successful environment for yourself.

Periods of calorie restriction—Regular periods of caloric restriction and fasting can support healthy blood sugars and lead to a reduced appetite. Committing yourself to a cleanse with only the consumption of clean plant-based foods and metabolic supportive additions such as ACV can really increase your likelihood of being successful.

Don't go out starving—Always consume something filling and healthy before an event where you know there will be decadent food and drinks available.

Prepare—This is one of the single most helpful tips; if that healthy meal is ready or premade or you have the ingredients already, then you will go straight to it rather than reaching for that easy, unhealthy snack or convenient meal.

Avoid eating after dinner—Anything you eat after your last meal is going straight to your fat stores. Instead, consume an herbal tea that is naturally sweet, such as licorice or a cinnamon-spice blend.

Set realistic goals—This is more likely to keep you motivated. Make it about how you feel rather than how much you weigh.

Don't eat too close to bedtime—Leave 3–4 hours between the last bite of dinner and the time your head hits the pillow. This helps you digest your meal.

Resistant Starch

How a special fiber called "resistant starch" supports weight control

Another important fiber that deserves a mention is called resistant starch. This type of fiber has been found to support good bacterial health and a healthy weight.

Our digestive system cannot digest or breakdown resistant starch, but when it reaches the large intestine (colon), it is broken down and fermented by the bacteria in the large bowel. This essentially acts as a food for the good guys.

How resistant starch supports weight loss

One of the reasons this fiber is so beneficial is because it helps us lose weight and maintain a healthy weight. Resistant starch helps to reduce hunger levels and increases satiety with fewer calories than other starches. Foods high in resistant starch work to support and maintain healthy gut microbiome. Resistant starch supports glycemic effects by improving insulin sensitity and blood sugar control. A 2012 study in the Journal of Nutrition demonstrated that consuming 15-30 g of resistant starch each day improved insulin sensitivity in overweight and obese subjects up to 50%. Not only this, but resistant starch reduces the rate of fat storage and increases fat oxidation, particularly after weight loss.

Foods high in resistant starch are unripe (green) bananas, plantains, legumes (particularly white beans, black beans, chickpeas, green peas, lentils, and kidney beans), cashews, oats, oatmeal, pearl barley, rice, yams, and potatoes. These foods may be cooked, but they must be cooled before they are consumed to be high in resistant starch. They must be consumed in their whole form, unprocessed only, to gain these benefits.

Body Mass Index (BMI)

BMI is another tool to determine if you are at a healthy weight. This number is calculated using a person's height and weight. BMI is considered to be a reliable way to estimate a person's body fat. BMI is currently used as the "gold standard" to screen for a person's risk of disease or death based on their weight category. Guidelines in the United States for a healthy waist circumference are less than 31–34 inches for women and 37–40 inches for men. When your waist measurements are greater than this suggestion, you're at an increased risk for diabetes, heart disease, and fatty liver disease.

Calculating BMI in Pounds and Feet

BMI = (weight in pounds × 4.88) / (height in feet × height in feet)

A person is 5'6" tall and has a weight of 160 lbs.
BMI = (160 × 4.88) / (5.5 × 5.5) = 25.81

Calculating BMI in Kilos

BMI = (bodyweight in kg) / (height in meters × height in meters)

Another person is 175 cm and has a weight of 70 kg
BMI = 70 / (1.75 × 1.75) = 22.86

BMI	Weight Status
Below 18.5	Underweight
18.5–24.9	Normal
25.0–29.9	Overweight
30.0 and Above	Obese

The negative aspect of using the BMI is that it doesn't cover all aspects of someone's individual stature so it will be incorrect for a very muscular person, or a thin person who has an unhealthy potbelly, and it doesn't indicate all potential health risks. It also doesn't account for the effects of age, sex, and race.

The best way to determine someone's health risks is to look at all the factors, including lifestyle habits, waist circumference, eating patterns, alcohol consumption, cigarette smoking, cardiovascular health, and blood sugar risk factors, to name a few.

Weight Loss Maintenance

It's one thing to lose weight, but it is another to maintain a healthy weight. People often find this to be much harder. They follow a set list of instructions, and then slowly find themselves falling back into long-term habits that send them right back to where they started. Any dietary plan that aims for weight loss will have to have some restrictions. Those that are put into place are often beneficial for stimulating hormonal changes that burn fat and reduce the appetite.

But if people find themselves slowly adding in too many not so healthy meals and snacks, then they are likely to find themselves exactly where they started.

Weight yo-yoing can be a very frustrating journey for anyone. Do you spend a lot of time thinking about your weight, analyzing everything you eat, and wondering what you are doing wrong? With this book I want to encourage long-term healthy eating habits, and I want to pass on what I know works for people who want to relearn how to stabilize a healthy weight and stay there. Losing weight is one thing, but I want readers and my patients to reach their goal weight and maintain it long-term. Cleanse plans are excellent starting points to dive into a long-term healthy eating plan; it's a way to rip off the bandage of unhealthy habits and get on with positive steps toward a healthy new you.

Tips for weight maintenance based on research

Eat at regular times—This helps you avoid skipping meals and getting too hungry! When people eat sporadically, they tend to make high-calorie choices that are convenient rather than healthy. This is a classic example of how people start falling back into old habits. Lack of preparation and skipping suggested meals and snacks could set you up for bad choices later on.

Watch your weight—but not too closely. It has been shown that when people weigh themselves regularly (about once or twice per week), it can help to keep them on track. But if you weigh yourself too often, it can become counterproductive, as hydration, hormones, stool motions, and other factors can affect your weight on a daily basis.

Eat loads of fruits and vegetables—which are filling, provide a myriad of nutrients, and have a low-calorie content overall. Filling up on fruits and vegetables is highly correlated with an increase in successful weight loss and maintenance.

Spend less time watching TV (and other screens)—We eat more when we sit staring at movies, games, shows, and social media. Studies show that people who lose weight and keep it off are more likely to watch LESS TV. One study at the Department of Psychology at The State University of New York at Geneseo found that people who are successful at maintaining weight loss over the long-term are more likely to spend a minimal amount of time watching TV.

Maintain a supportive network—It has been shown that if we have healthy friends, we are more likely to be healthy. So why not get healthy together? Having the right support around you can make all the difference in the world. Health professionals, counseling, family, and friends, along with health-focused communities and groups, are all great places to find support and camaraderie.

Support yourself emotionally in all ways—Emotional eating can hinder someone's health plan. See more on emotional eating in the previous "Emotional Eating" section.

Prepare—Make food ahead of time, store healthy meals in the freezer, and learn a few recipes that are quick and easy. Always stock your pantry and fridge with a few basic healthy essential items.

Get 7–9 hours of sleep—People who get less than 7 hours of sleep per night are more likely to be overweight and struggle with cravings and episodes of overeating.

Get moving—People who move their bodies every day, even if it's just mild to moderate exercise for 30–60 minutes, were more likely to maintain a healthy weight.

How to Incorporate ACV into Meals and Recipes

Apple cider vinegar not only makes a great salad dressing, but it can also be used in other recipes, such as curries, stews, soups, bone broths, vegetable broths, and seafood broths, to help extract the nutrients into the water. It is an excellent tasty meat-marinating ingredient, as it helps to penetrate the skin and infuse the other ingredient flavors of the marinade into the meat.

When added to soups, ACV can add a bright flavor that brings out the other flavors. You can add it at the end of the cooking time or earlier, depending on your preference.

It can be a great addition to rice before cooking to give it extra fluffiness. Adding it to sauces and chutneys will add a tangy element.

It can add a really tangy flavor to juices and smoothies, although I would add it in very small amounts to find your happy place.

Apple cider vinegar does not spoil, as it is a preservative in itself. Thus adding it to food that needs to be stored can help preserve the food.

ACV can be a substitute for an acidic ingredient, such as lemon. Mixed with pepper and garlic, it will give a tangy taste to the food.

The Benefits of Healthful Probiotic Foods and Beverages

Fermented foods and probiotic drinks are all the rage at the moment. The studies that support and promote the regular consumption of healthy beneficial bacteria are proliferating. The studies on how a healthy microbiome has an immense impact on all areas of our health seem to be never ending. These are hugely exciting developments in nutritional research.

Probiotic foods include:

- Apple cider vinegar
- Other unpasteurized vinegars
- Sauerkraut, kimchi, and other fermented vegetables
- Kefir (organic dairy or non-dairy)
- Yogurt (organic dairy or non-dairy)
- Tempeh, miso, natto
- Kombucha

Each person is said to contain approximately 5 lbs. of bacteria, and this 5 lbs. of bacteria has an enormous effect on our health and well-being! It has been said that the microbiome behaves as another organ in the human body. Poor microbial health is associated with chronic health conditions, such as obesity, inflammatory bowel disease, depression, anxiety, infections, and poor immunity.

A healthy microbiome supports the:

- Digestion of food and the metabolism of essential nutrients
- Regulation of our immune system in our gut—we have more immune cells in our digestive system than everywhere else combined
- Responsiveness of the immune system
- Control of inflammatory mediators and hormone signaling
- Signaling of our brain's chemistry and mood

Microbial health has become implicated in autoimmune disease and other immune and inflammatory disorders, such as eczema, allergies, IBS, lactose intolerance, constipation, asthma, and other chronic health disorders. In some studies, it has been demonstrated that changing the environment of the gut microbiome in mice positively impacts asthma and other chronic immune diseases, reduces their severity, and in some cases, reverses them completely. **Vinegar was also used in these studies to encourage the positive microbial change, with very strong results.**

Research has also shown in mice studies that the lack of fermentable fibers and, therefore, lack of good bacteria in our diets may pave the way for allergic inflammatory diseases. Mice that were fed a high-fiber diet had increased circulating levels of short-chain fatty acids (SCFAs) and were protected against allergic inflammation in the lung. Conversely, a low-fiber diet increased allergic airway disease. The types of fibers that support healthy microbial health are predominantly soluble fibers that are still present in freshly made juices and other whole foods.

Foods that are high in fiber that support the production of SCFAs in the bowel are berries, apples, pears, figs, green beans, broccoli, spinach, dandelion greens, leek, garlic, asparagus, Brussels sprouts, cauliflower, and root vegetables, such as sweet potatoes, onions, and carrots.

What environmental influences negatively affect our gut health?

- Overconsumption of processed foods versus natural whole foods
- Limited microbial exposure and outdoor time: reduced exposure to the outdoors, animals, plants, soil and other outside organisms
- Overly hygienic environments: chlorinated water supplies, hand sanitizers, anti-microbial cleaners, antibacterial hand-washes, and our overwashed and hygienic food items (historically people consumed soil microorganisms in their food from underwashed produce)
- Some medication: antibiotics, NSAIDs, antacid medications, oral contraceptives
- Possible farming contaminates: pesticides, herbicides, chemical fertilizers
- Antibiotics used in conventional farming
- Alcohol
- High-sugar diets
- Food pasteurization

Factors that positively influence our gut bacteria are prebiotics, which are the foods that feed the good guys! The most common naturally occurring prebiotics are inulins, fructooligosaccharides (FOS), and galactooligosaccharides (GOS), all of which pass through the digestive system without being digested or absorbed. Foods rich in prebiotics include asparagus, artichokes, leeks, onions, garlic, bananas, whole grains, legumes, cruciferous vegetables, and leafy greens.

A very important long-term pattern to follow is to consume more fruits and vegetables, juices, smoothies, and other whole foods. You should also include apple cider vinegar and other fermented foods and drinks that will have a very strong impact on your long-term gut health, your immune health, and your weight. These are the most positive steps you can take toward supporting your gut microbiome, weight, and health.

Sleep to Lose

Studies have shown that when we sleep for the recommended amount of 7–9 hours a night, our weight loss may be more significant. People who are deprived of sleep are more likely to feel hungry and have increased cravings due to feelings of fatigue, tiredness, and hormonal changes.

Deep, restful, high-quality sleep plays an important role in cell and tissue renewal, repair, and hormonal health. Sleepless nights are normally followed by a day where, no matter what a person eats, they still feel hungry. This is due to the hormonal changes that occur in leptin and ghrelin. Ghrelin, which is produced in the stomach and pancreas, stimulates appetite and promotes fat retention, while leptin, produced in the fat cells, sends a signal to the brain that we are full.

A study published in the *American Journal of Clinical Nutrition* in 2011 showed that sleep-deprived participants felt hungrier than the group who had significant sleep, and the sleep-deprived participants had higher levels of ghrelin (hungry hormone) and lower levels of leptin (satiety hormone). Insufficient sleep can also cause the release of the stress hormone cortisol, which can stimulate hunger.

At the 2006 American Thoracic Society International Conference, it was shown that women who slept 5 hours per night or less were 32% more likely to experience major weight gain (an increase of 33 lbs. or more) and 15% more likely to become obese over the course of the 16-year study, compared to those who slept 7 hours a night. The women who slept 6 hours per night were still 12% more likely to experience major weight gain and 6% more likely to become obese, compared to women who slept 7 hours a night.

There is also evidence that less sleep may increase the expression of obesity-related genes or that the longer periods of sleep suppress these genes. These genes affect how the body uses energy, our metabolic health, how fat is stored, and the feeling of being satisfied after a meal.

Other studies have indicated that with less sleep you may lose more muscle when weight loss occurs, and with increased sleep more fat is lost during weight loss. Inadequate sleep interferes with the body's ability to metabolize carbohydrates and causes high blood sugar levels and increased insulin levels (fat-storing hormone). It drives down leptin levels, which increases carbohydrate cravings, and reduces levels of the human growth hormone (HGH), which helps to regulate fat and muscle. These all can lead to an increased risk of diabetes, heart disease, high blood pressure, and other chronic health conditions. It is also important to note that too much sleep can be counterproductive and increase weight gains. So, remember to turn in early to support weight control and weight loss.

Benefits of Exercise for Weight Loss and Health

This is the stuff that makes you young and keeps you agile! As we discussed in the section on weight maintenance, exercise that is consistent and regular will certainly help you to lose the weight, but more importantly, it will help you to keep it off!

Weight loss and maintenance
Exercise boosts the metabolism for longer periods throughout the day, thus allowing greater calorie burn to help weight loss and maintenance. Exercise speeds the rate of energy use, resulting in an increased metabolic rate.

Mood
Exercise stimulates various brain chemicals that may leave you feeling happier and more relaxed. It has been shown to be as effective as some antidepressants. It may take at least 30 minutes of exercise a day for at least 3–5 days a week to significantly improve symptoms of depression. It was shown in one study at the Duke University Medical Center in Durham, NC

that after 16 weeks of treatment, exercise was as effective in reducing depression among patients with major depressive disorder as medication.

Energy
Regular physical activity can improve your muscle strength and boost your endurance. Exercise and physical activity deliver oxygen and nutrients to your tissues and help your cardiovascular system work more efficiently.

Better sleep
Exercise certainly supports better sleep, as exercise physically tires the body and improves sleep depth and length.

Improved cognition and memory
Exercise has been shown to help stimulate new brain cells and improve memory. Researchers at the Institute of Basic Medical Sciences, National Cheng Kung University Medical College in Tainan, Taiwan, have found that the area of the brain that is stimulated by exercise is responsible for memory and learning.

Longevity
Exercise increases your life expectancy and reduces your risk of dying prematurely. In one long-term study that was conducted at the Ostra University Hospital in Sweden, it was demonstrated that exercise offers some protection against mortality from heart disease, cancer, and other causes.

Muscle health
Studies have repeatedly shown that strength training increases muscle mass and decreases fat tissue. Increased muscle mass increases caloric burn.

Bone strength
Being active has a positive impact on bone health. Regular weight-bearing exercise promotes bone formation, delays bone loss, and may protect against bone loss associated with aging.

It's medically proven that people who do regular physical activity have:

- 35% lower risk of coronary heart disease and stroke
- 50% lower risk of type 2 diabetes
- 50% lower risk of colon cancer
- 20% lower risk of breast cancer
- 30% lower risk of early death
- 83% lower risk of osteoarthritis
- 68% lower risk of hip fracture
- 30% lower risk of falls (among older adults)
- 30% lower risk of depression
- 30% lower risk of dementia

Suggested exercises

Walking is a great place to start. Try walking in the fresh air and somewhere that is enjoyable. Put on some great tunes and move! This will improve your health results and changes during the 7-Day Cleanse and beyond.

Other fun activities—gym workouts, swimming, yoga, Pilates, spin, cycling, physical labor, house cleaning, dancing, hiking, and jogging are all great ways to get active.

Other helpful tips—To get active, you can take the stairs instead of the elevator, park the car a little further away from where you want to go, or hop off the train or bus one stop earlier, so your walk home is a little longer. Any type of incidental exercise that you partake in will add up and make a difference in the long-term.

The most important point to remember is to make it fun, so you are more likely to stick to it on a consistent basis.

It's important to note that weight loss is 80% diet and 20% exercise!

If you have a serious medical condition before starting this cleanse, it is recommended that you consult your doctor.

Macronutrients for Good Health and Weight Control

PROTEIN

What is protein?

Protein is found throughout the body—in muscle, bone, skin, hair, and virtually every other body part or tissue. You also use protein to make enzymes, hormones, and other body chemicals. Protein is an important building block of bones, muscles, cartilage, skin, and blood.

You need protein in your diet to help your body repair cells and make new ones. Protein is also important for growth and development in children, teens, and pregnant women.

Along with fat and carbohydrates, protein is a macronutrient, meaning that the body needs relatively large amounts of it. Vitamins and minerals, which are needed in only small quantities, are called micronutrients.

Protein-rich foods are broken down into amino acids during digestion. The human body needs a number of amino acids in large amounts to maintain good health.

Protein on your cleanse

The ACV Cleanse is a short-term plan that is designed to help you jump into healthier eating habits and kick-start permanent health changes. The average protein intake from your 7-Day ACV Cleanse is approximately 20–30 g per day. For a very short period of time it is completely fine and healthy to reduce your protein and your calories to enhance your health and jump-start a healthier lifestyle. After the Cleanse, it's important to get enough protein and amino acids.

Protein requirements after your cleanse

The recommended daily allowance (RDA) of protein established by the Institute of Medicine (IOM) is 0.36 g of protein per pound of body weight (0.8 g of protein per kilo of body weight). This is a minimum guideline for sedentary adults. So for example, the average sedentary woman requires 46 g of protein per day, while the average sedentary man requires 56 g per day. Include moderate to higher intensity exercise and it moves up to 0.45–0.55 g per pound of body weight (1–1.2 g per kilo of body weight).

The National Health and Nutrition Examination Survey found that the average American male consumes 102 grams of protein per day and the average female eats about 70 grams.

The issue with these basic calculations is that they don't take into account difference in body fat and muscle composition between individuals, which can vary considerably between two people who weigh the same but have different percentages of body fat and lean muscle. The serving sizes we have become accustomed to also complicate the matter. An idea amount of meat-based protein for most people would be a 3–4 oz. serving of meat—not a 9 or 12 oz. steak!

An overweight man who does little exercise weighs 175 lbs. and has a high body fat composition at 25%. Compare that to a lean man who has a low body fat index of 12% and also weighs 175 lbs. These two people have very different protein requirements.

Protein requirements calculation:

Weight lbs. × (1–body fat %) = lean mass × 0.45 g
= Protein amount required

Example 1: A women with a body fat composition of 25% and a weight of 150 lbs. would determine her protein requirement in the following way:

150 × (1–0.25) = 112.5 × 0.45
= 51 g of protein per day

Example 2: A man with a higher muscle mass who has a body fat composition of 10%, weighs 210 lbs., and works out at a high intensity would calculate his requirements as follows:

Weight lbs. × (1–body fat %) = lean mass × 0.55 g = Protein amount required

210 × (1–0.10) = 189 × 0.55
= 104 g of protein per day

Example 3: A man weighs 210 lbs, has a body fat composition of 25%, and is lightly to moderately active. He would determine his protein needs as:

Weight lbs. × (1–body fat %) = lean mass × 0.45 g = Protein amount required

210 × (1–0.25) = 157.5 × 0.45
= 71 g of protein per day

So, as you can see from these three examples protein needs vary based on muscle composition and activity level, even for people with the same weight.

To work out kilos (kg), simply convert kilos × 2.2 = pounds

This calculation is more accurate when you are looking at somebody with a large fat composition. The United States is said to have the highest protein intake in the world, along with other Western countries, such as Australia, which are not far behind.

Protein requirements are increased during pregnancy, for athletes, and for seniors. Protein needs are also increased for people with injuries, people who are post-surgery or in recovery, and people with other tissue repair situations. The requirement increases by approximately 25%. This will ensure that a protein deficiency does not occur.

Protein content of food:

Red meat, pork, and poultry average 5–9 g of protein per ounce.

Protein content per 4 oz. cooked

- Chicken breast—32 g
- Lamb—28 g
- Beef—28 g
- Salmon—28 g
- Snapper—28 g
- Pork—24 g

Eggs contain about 6–8 g of protein per egg

Seeds and nuts contain on average 5–10 g of protein per ¼ cup

Protein content per ¼ cup

- Pumpkin seeds–10 g
- Macadamia nuts–3 g
- Almonds–7.5 g
- Cashews–6 g
- Pistachios–8 g

Cooked legumes average about 7–8 g per half cup

Protein content per ½ cup, cooked

- Lentils–15.6 g
- Kidney–14.4 g
- Split peas–16 g
- Adzuki–17 g
- Tempeh 3 oz.–19 g

Cooked grains average 5–7 g per cup

Protein content per ½ cup, cooked

- Rice, brown–2.5 g
- Quinoa–4 g
- Buckwheat–5.7 g
- Whole-wheat spaghetti–7 g
- Rye bread, 1 slice–3 g

Vegetables average 1–2 g per cup

Protein content per 1 cup, cooked

- Kale–4 g
- Spinach–5 g
- Broccoli–4 g
- Asparagus–4 g
- Artichokes–4 g

Other high-protein plant foods

In addition to the foods listed above, a few others deserve a special mention for their protein content. They can be easily added to juices, smoothies, and other meals to up the plant protein.

Hemp seeds (hemp hearts): About 33% protein, providing 11 g per 3 tablespoons; they also contain all 20 amino acids in an easily digestible form and are loaded with omega-3 fats.

Spirulina: 70% protein by weight; 4 g of protein per 2 teaspoon serving; contains 18 of the amino acids and all of the essentials and is easily assimilated.

Sprouts: The quality of the protein and the fiber content of beans, nuts, seeds, and grains improves when sprouted.

Bee pollen: 40% protein and one of nature's most complete foods, it's an excellent addition for variety.

SUGAR AND CARBOHYDRATES

Carbohydrates are important for long-term health, but it is important to distinguish between healthy carbs and not so healthy carbs. When I promote good health, the carbohydrates I encourage are fruits and vegetables, nuts, seeds, some whole grains, and legumes. This doesn't include processed carbohydrates, such as breads, bagels, breakfast cereals, crackers, biscuits, white pasta, and sweets that we typically associate with carbs. These are common high-processed foods that are stripped of their nutrients and fiber.

Unfortunately, most people eat the types of carbohydrates that are convenient and convert into sugar very quickly. This exacerbates blood sugar irregularities, weight gain, and fatigue.

Fresh fruits and vegetables are loaded with nutrients that support good health and help to support healthy blood sugar. 50–75% of your plate should be colored food, particularly the low-starch kind, at least twice daily or more.

BLOOD SUGAR

The problem with elevated blood sugar that comes from eating high glycemic carbohydrate-rich foods is that it switches off your satiety hormones and stimulates and increases your hungry hormones. This drives increased fat storage, especially belly fat.

Excess insulin is produced in response to high blood sugar and signals the liver to store fat, creates cellular inflammation as a type of stress response, raises triglycerides, disrupts other blood fats, increases blood pressure, and disrupts other hormones. It also increases the appetite and cravings for more sweet and starchy foods, thus creating an unhealthy pattern that can be hard to get out of. Doesn't sound good, does it?

All of this is caused by the foods that spike our blood sugar! After all of these changes occur metabolically, the fatigue, lethargy, and cravings will hit. Sound fun? I think not.

This is where a healthy plan such as the ACV plan can help you to curb these addictions and move into a long-term healthy eating pattern to balance and support a healthy metabolism. It's like ripping the bandage off in one swoop!

Sugar also causes premature aging both inside and out! If you want to look good and keep those wrinkles away, then sugar isn't for you.

NOT ALL CALORIES ARE CREATED EQUAL

The amount of people I've seen who follow this rule still surprises me. This can set people up to form really unhealthy eating patterns; some people believe a biscuit is equivalent to an apple, so they might as well eat the biscuit. The body metabolizes these foods completely differently and they have very different effects on your hormones, energy, and metabolic health.

The biscuit creates inflammation, a sugar spike, and increased fat-storing hormone production, while the apple stabilizes blood sugar, provides nutrients and fiber, and reduces inflammation. The nutrients and fiber regulate the appetite, which reduces cravings and supports successful weight loss. But yes, the apple and the biscuit do have the same amount of calories.

VEGETABLE AND FRUIT CONSIDERATIONS—WHAT TO EAT MORE OF, AND LESS OF, FOR WEIGHT LOSS

Fruits and vegetables differ in their dietary fiber and carbohydrate composition. The types of fruits and vegetables that a person consumes play a strong role in his or her ability to lose weight. Lower glycemic fruits and vegetables have a stronger influence on maintaining healthy blood sugar levels, which have an impact on weight and appetite control.

PLOS Medicine released a study that analyzed 134,000 people over a 24-year period. It showed a very strong link between a high intake of fruits and vegetables with increased weight loss and healthy weight maintenance, although some fruits and vegetables were not linked to weight loss. There was an association between consuming a higher intake of starchy vegetables, including corn, peas, and potatoes, with an associated weight gain, while consuming lower glycemic fruits and vegetable had a strong weight loss correlation.

There was a reported emphasis on successful weight loss in participants consuming more:

- Berries
- Apples
- Pears
- Cauliflower

- Broccoli
- Spinach
- Kale
- Radishes

- Swiss chard
- Collard greens
- Rutabaga
- Turnips

Eat freely

Eat lots of vegetable for increased weight loss. Vegetables to eat freely include spinach, kale, watercress, lettuces, endive, chicory, green beans, rainbow chard, celery, cucumber, asparagus, cabbage, bok choy, arugula (rocket), mushrooms, zucchini, bamboo shoots, fennel, cauliflower, leek, radicchio, bell peppers, and Brussels sprouts.

Moderate amounts of these

Limit your intake of starchy cooked vegetables, such as potatoes, corn, peas, and sweet potatoes. This means that you should eat them if you like them, just not in massive portions, since even the healthiest foods and meals can impact your weight if eaten in excessive quantities.

When eating grains, it's best to keep them to a smaller portion. Grains can increase your blood sugar if eaten in larger amounts.

Consider sticking with only whole grains, such as quinoa, buckwheat, amaranth, black (wild) rice, or any other ancient whole grain, and prepare them properly to increase their digestibility. This also applies to other starchy whole foods, such as legumes. Eating certain types of healthy food in too large quantities may inhibit your weight loss.

BASIC PORTION SIZES FOR WEIGHT CONTROL:

- Nuts: ½ cup
- Grains (amaranth, buckwheat, rice, quinoa, millet, etc.): ½ cup, cooked
- Rolled oats: 1 cup, cooked
- Oil: 1 tablespoon
- Nut butter: 1 tablespoon

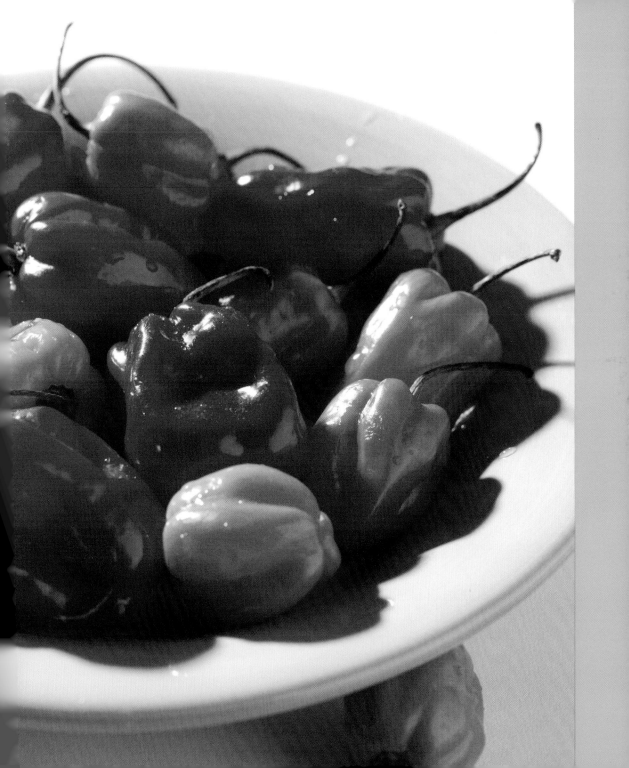

- Beans, lentils, and split peas: ½ cup, cooked
- Fruit—varies depending on variety, 2–4 servings depending on sweetness
- Vegetables—eat freely, particularly the low glycemic kind
- Potatoes, corn, and peas—½–1 cup
- Animal-based protein—4 oz. cooked fish, meat, or poultry. Another great guide is to use your whole flat hand for fish, mid knuckles and palm for chicken, and palm size only for red meat.

This is a general guide. Needs may vary for each individual.

WHAT'S THE FAT ON FAT?

For many years, people have been fat-phobic due to the stream of fad diets claiming that fats make you fat. Low-fat diets claim to reduce the risk of various diseases. With all this misinformation, many people started eating far too many carbohydrates in the way of processed grains to help them fill up. Because fat is extremely filling (and the most satisfying of all the macronutrients), we created a nutritional hole in our diets. This misinformation led people to increased weight problems, diabetes, obesity, and heart problems.

Just like not all carbs or calories are equal, not all fat is equal. It's important to identify which are the slimming fats and which are not!

Natural fats in the diet increase the production and stimulation of hormones that tell you to stop eating and increase your appetite satiety. But this doesn't mean that healthy fats can be eaten in unlimited amounts.

Fat is important for hormone regulation, satiety, appetite control, weight loss, vitamin D synthesis, absorption of fat-soluble vitamins, reduced cardiovascular disease, healthy bones, healthy brain and nerve function, and a strong immune system.

If you are not eating enough essential fats in the diet, you are more likely to suffer from:

- Poor concentration
- Fatigue
- Lethargy
- Feeling full but still being hungry

- Wanting something sweet after a full meal
- Mid-afternoon energy drops
- Dry, itchy, scaling, or flaking skin
- Soft, cracked, or brittle nails
- Hard earwax
- Tiny bumps on the backs of your arms or torso
- Achy, stiff joints

Foods that contain healthy fat:

All these fats and oils are recommended as unrefined and cold pressed—olive oil, avocado oil, coconut oil, macadamia oil, grass-fed organic ghee, and butter. Healthy fats, like omega-3 fats found in wild salmon, are also found in other foods, such as avocado, oily fish, nuts, and seeds.

- Nuts—walnuts, macadamia nuts, pecans, pine nuts, almonds, cashews, and hazelnuts
- Oily fish—sardines, mackerel, herring, and wild salmon
- Seeds—pumpkin, sesame, chia, hemp, and sunflower

Saturated fat—Saturated fats have been given more of a pass in recent times. When eating meat, it is best to consume organic and grass-fed whenever possible to reduce the toxic load on our bodies and to ensure healthier fat content. Conventional grain-fed meats tend to have a higher fat rancidity with increased marbling, and the fat often contains pollutants that the animal has been exposed to.

The most toxic fats of all are:

Trans-fats—These are mostly made to extend the shelf life of baked foods. They have been found to cause a long list of health problems, such as infertility, cardiovascular disease, and obesity (to name a few). They are often listed as vegetable fats, hydrogenated vegetable oils, partially hydrogenated vegetable oils, or margarine. Crisps, chocolate, spreads, pastries, and other processed packaged foods contain trans-fats.

Processed vegetable oils—Highly refined GMO oils can wreak havoc on the body by stimulating inflammatory pathways, which contribute to all diseases in the body.

Take-home message

Healthy fats help you stay slim and support a healthy metabolism.

More on food allergies and intolerances that may be affecting your health:

Food allergies and food intolerances can be difficult to diagnose: even when scratch testing, patch testing, and blood testing are used, it is still difficult to identify all food allergies and intolerances. Avoiding any suspected food and re-introducing it after a period of time is a great way to determine if the food is the culprit in causing any health-related problems.

Common food allergens:

It is believed that 4–8% of people in developed countries have at least 1 food allergy. Common reactions to food allergens range from mild to severe and can include itchiness, urticaria, eczema, swelling, difficulty swallowing, hoarse voice, wheezing, light-headedness, drop in blood pressure, sneezing, asthma, nasal congestion, nausea, vomiting, diarrhea, abdominal pain, bloating, fatigue, or other digestive problems.

Gluten—Gluten intolerance is caused by an immunological reaction to gluten, which is found in wheat, rye, barley, spelt, and kamut.

Dairy foods—Dairy foods can cause problems due to their proteins and/or lactose content. Dairy foods include yogurt, milk, creams, cheeses, butter, ice cream and packaged foods. These can be cow, sheep, and/or goat dairy.

Soy foods—Soy products, including soy milk, soy cheese, tofu, soy sauce, TVP, soy flour, meat substitutes, and miso can cause allergic reactions. Read nutrition labels, as soy can sometimes be used as a filler or bulking agent in many food products.

Eggs—Egg allergy symptoms usually occur a few minutes to a few hours after eating eggs or foods containing eggs.

Peanuts— Peanuts are found in muesli/granola bars, mixes, cakes, bars, packaged foods and many other places. It's important to be aware that anaphylaxis may occur in peanut allergy.

Note: Allergies can develop to any food, since the proteins in the foods primarily stimulate an immunological response.

Food Intolerances—Food intolerance tends to develop over time and may be caused by repeated consumption. It is a little more difficult to diagnose, as it can be due to repeated exposure rather than a reaction that occurs after only one exposure.

GLUTEN

Gluten intolerance is a highly controversial topic, and there are many reasons why grains containing gluten are becoming more of a problem for many people. I want to mention gluten as a topic since, as a clinician, I have seen many health problems improve with the exclusion of gluten.

Celiac Disease

When people with celiac disease (CD) eat wheat, the immune system in their gut mistakenly identifies the gluten proteins as foreign invaders and mounts an attack. The immune system doesn't attack only the gluten proteins; it also attacks the gut lining itself, leading to degeneration of the intestinal lining, leaky gut, massive inflammation, and other harmful effects. People with this type of CD are the most severely affected group and account for approximately 1% of the population, but severe CD is on the rise, particularly in the elderly. In one study, after 45 years of follow-up, undiagnosed CD was associated with a nearly 4-fold increased risk of death. The prevalence of undiagnosed CD seems to have increased dramatically in the United States during the past 50 years. It is estimated that 80% of people with CD have no idea that they have it. Many people who have CD may not have any digestive or abdominal symptoms but suffer from anemia, fatigue, muscle soreness, or other associated symptoms. It is recommended that you be tested for CD if you have the following symptoms:

- Gastrointestinal and classical symptoms: diarrhea, weight loss, abdominal distention, failure to thrive
- Autoimmune diseases: type 1 diabetes, thyroid disorders, Sjögren's syndrome, microscopic colitis, inflammatory bowel disease, etc.
- Elevated liver enzymes
- Iron-deficiency anemia
- Osteoporosis
- Delayed puberty

- Infertility
- Irritable bowel syndrome
- First-degree relatives with CD

Gluten Sensitivity

The other group of people that may be affected by gluten are classified as having non-celiac gluten sensitivity (NCGS). This is a new classification that some do not accept, but studies are suggesting it is correct. Interestingly, just 30 years ago celiac disease was not accepted as a legitimate disease. Today, it is mostly diagnosed by the elimination of gluten from the diet. If gluten is reintroduced, the symptoms reoccur. It is estimated that NCGS occurs in approximately 6–8% of the population, based on anti-gliadin antibodies in blood tests.

Problems associated with NCGS that are not gut-related are fatigue, muscle aches, depression, autoimmune diseases, eczema, psoriasis, arthritis, hives, and other inflammatory conditions.

The consumption of dwarf wheat may contribute to the increase in immune and digestive problems that are often attributed to gluten. Grains and legumes that have been traditionally harvested through soaking, fermenting, and sprouting produce more bio-available nutrients and help to reduce lectin content. Dwarf wheat is produced with a greater annual yield than these smaller-yield ancient grains, which results in fewer nutrients. This practice is cheaper and more efficient for the manufacturer.

Other Possible Causes of Gluten Sensitivity

- A higher presence of Glia-9 in modern wheat, which is the type of gluten most associated with health problems.
- In some cases gluten is blamed where FODMAPs (Fermentable Oligosaccharides, Disaccharides, Monosaccharides and Polyols) are the issue, particularly in cases of IBS.
- To reduce the wear-and-tear on machinery, some manufactures saturate the wheat with glycosphate (Roundup®) prior to harvesting (called "desiccation").
- Newer wheat varieties, such as the dwarf wheat, have a higher gluten content to improve the consistency and sponginess of baked goods

- Gluten acts as a natural insecticide, so farmers favor higher gluten varieties, which are more likely to cause health problems
- Higher consumption over the years of wheat-based products

Some studies indicate einkorn and other older wheat grain varieties are associated with fewer health problems and may not stimulate any health issues at all. These findings indicate that modern wheat has a unique ability to trigger an auto-immune reaction in the gut and is probably the main reason why celiac disease and gluten sensitivity are on the rise.

MORE ON LEGUMES

Beans, split peas, and lentils are excellent sources of fiber, protein, vitamins, and minerals. For some people, they can be difficult to digest and may need to be avoided, particularly in cases of digestive disorders like IBS, increased gut permeability (aka "leaky gut"), indigestion, and excessive flatulence. For others, when prepared correctly, legumes can be an excellent source of nutrients.

Soaking, rinsing, toasting and cooking legumes all reduce the prevalence of anti-nutrients. Traditionally, legumes (particularly beans) have been soaked in water, rinsed, and re-soaked to deactivate the digestive irritants. It is also advisable to cook legumes at high temperatures to help deactivate the anti-nutrients.

Anti-nutrients include phytates, lectins, protease inhibitors, tannins, and oxalates. Soaking the legumes can reduce them by 13–50%, as they are mostly water-soluble. Cooking, sprouting, and fermenting the legumes further deactivates these compounds. This increases the bioavailability of the nutrients for improved absorption and can reduce digestive upset in some people.

When preparing legumes, try to incorporate these preparation guidelines; if they still cause any digestive upset, then they may be best avoided for the time being.

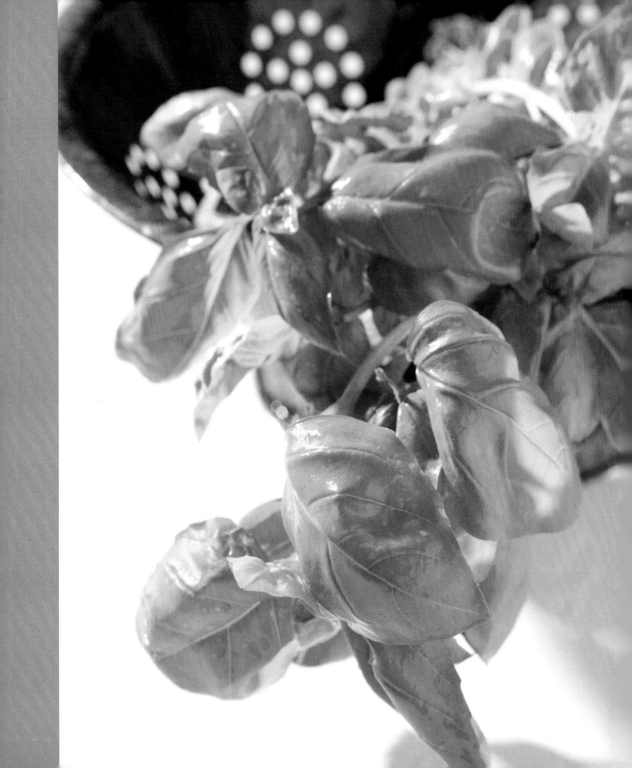

Claire Georgiou B.HSc (C. Med) ND MATMS is an Australian naturopath, herbalist, and nutritionist with a Bachelor of Health Science in Comparative Medicine. She has more than 14 years of clinical experience specializing in liver disease, weight loss programs, autoimmune disease, thyroid conditions, diabetes, insulin resistance, digestive disorders, chronic infections, children's health, and fertility. Claire has worked closely with Dr. Sandra Cabot—"The Liver Doctor"—for many years, and she is one of the nutritionists who runs the Guided Reboot programs on the enormously popular website Reboot with Joe (www.rebootwithjoe.com), writing health-related articles and creating healthy recipes. Claire consults in private practice in Sydney and also offers consults out of area.

You can find Claire at her website: www.healthyyouliving.com.au

References

Allday, E, "100 Trillion Good Bacteria Call the Human Body Home," *SF Gate*. Hearst Communications. 5 July 2012. http://www.sfgate.com/health/article/100-trillion-good-bacteria-call-human-body-home-3683153.php

"Amazing Apple Cider Vinegar," *Healthline*. Healthline Media. 3 May 2013. http://www.healthline.com/health/amazing-apple-cider-vinegar#3

Bao W, Li K, Rong S, Yao P, Hao L, Ying C, Zhang X, Nussler A, Liu L, "Curcumin alleviates ethanol-induced hepatocytes oxidative damage involving heme oxygenase-1 induction," *Journal of Ethnopharmacology*, 2010 Mar 24;128(2):549-53. doi: 10.1016/j.jep.2010.01.029. Epub 2010 Jan 18.

Bertoia M, Mukamal K, Cahill L, Hou T, Ludwig D, Mozaffarian D, Willett W, Hu F, Rimm E, "Changes in Intake of Fruits and Vegetables and Weight Change in United States Men and Women Followed for Up to 24 Years: Analysis from Three Prospective Cohort Studies," *PLOS Medicine*, 22 Sept 2015. doi: 10.1371/journal.pmed.1001878

Beheshti Z , Chan YH, Sharif Nia H, Hajihosseini F, Nazari R, Shaabani M, Taghi Salehi Omran M. "Influence of apple cider vinegar on blood lipids." Life Science Journal. 2012;9(4):2431-2440.

Blumenthal JA, Babyak MA, Moore KA, Craighead WE, Herman S, Khatri P, Waugh R, Napolitano MA, Forman LM, Appelbaum M, Doraiswamy PM, Krishnan KR, "Effects of exercise training on older patients with major depression," *Archives of Internal Medicine*. 1999 Oct 25;159(19):2349-56.

Boschmann M, Steiniger J, Franke G, Birkenfeld A, Luft F, and Jordan J, "Water Drinking Induces Thermogenesis through Osmosensitive Mechanisms," *The Journal of Clinical Endocrinology & Metabolism* 2013; 92 (8). doi: http://dx.doi.org/10.1210/jc.2006-1438

Brighenti F, Benini L, Del Rio D, Casiraghi C, Pellegrini N, Scazzina F, Jenkins DJ, Vantini I, "Colonic fermentation of indigestible carbohydrates contributes to the second-meal effect," *American Journal of Clinical Nutrition*, 2006 Apr;83(4):817-22.

Budak N, Aykin E, Seydim A, Greene A, and Guzel-Seydim Z, "Functional Properties of Vinegar," *Journal of Food Science* .79, no. 5 (2014): R757-764, doi: 10.1111/1750-3841.12434

"Caffeine Content for Coffee, Tea, Soda, and More." *Mayo Clinic*. Mayo Foundation for Medical Education and Research. http://www.mayoclinic.org/healthy-lifestyle/nutrition-and-healthy-eating/in-depth/caffeine/art-20049372

Dennis EA, Dengo AL, Comber DL, Flack KD, Savla J, Davy KP, Davy BM, "Water consumption increases weight loss during a hypocaloric diet intervention in middle-aged and older adults," *Obesity (Silver Spring)*. 2010 Feb;18(2):300-7. doi: 10.1038/oby.2009.235. Epub 2009 Aug 6.

Di Sabatino A, Corazza GR, "Coeliac Disease," *Lancet*. 2009 Apr 25;373(9673):1480-93. doi: 10.1016/S0140-6736(09)60254-3

Dulloo AG, Duret C, Rohrer D, Girardier L, Mensi N, Fathi M, Chantre P, Vandermander J, "Efficacy of a green tea extract rich in catechin polyphenols and caffeine in increasing 24-h energy expenditure and fat oxidation in humans," *American Journal of Clinical Nutrition*, 1999 Dec;70(6):1040-5
http://www.ncbi.nlm.nih.gov/pubmed/10584049

Fan MS, Zhao FJ, Fairweather-Tait SJ, Poulton PR, Dunham SJ, McGrath SP, "Evidence of decreasing mineral density in wheat grain over the last 160 years," *Journal of Trace Elements in Medicine and Biology*, 2008;22(4):315-24. doi: 10.1016/j.jtemb.2008.07.002. Epub 2008 Sep 17.

Fasano A, Sapone A, Zevallos V, Schuppan D, "Nonceliac gluten sensitivity," *Gastroenterolog*, 2015 May;148(6):1195-204. doi: 10.1053/j.gastro.2014.12.049. Epub 2015 Jan 9

Feizizadeh S, Salehi-Abargouei A, Akbari V, "Efficacy and safety of *Saccharomyces boulardii* for acute diarrhea," *Pediatrics*, 2014; 134(1): e176-e191

"Fourth National Report on Human Exposure to Environmental Chemicals," *Centers for Disease Control*, 2009.
http://www.cdc.gov/exposurereport/pdf/FourthReport.pdf

Fushimi T, Suruga K, Oshima Y, Fukiharu M, Tsukamoto Y, Goda T, "Dietary acetic acid reduces serum cholesterol and triacylglycerols in rats fed a cholesterol-rich diet," *British Journal of Nutrition*. 2006 May;95(5):916-24
http://www.ncbi.nlm.nih.gov/pubmed/16611381

"Gut Reaction, Part 2," *Catalyst*. ABC. 21 Aug 2014.
http://www.abc.net.au/catalyst/stories/4070977.htm

Higgins JA, "Resistant starch and energy balance: impact on weight loss and maintenance," *Critical Reviews in Food Science and Nutrition*, 2014;54(9):1158-66. doi: 10.1080/10408398.2011.629352.

Johnston CS, Buller AJ, "Vinegar and peanut products as complementary foods to reduce postprandial glycemia," *Journal of the American Dietetic Association*, 2005 Dec;105(12):1939-42
http://www.ncbi.nlm.nih.gov/pubmed/16321601

Johnston CS, Steplewska I, Long CA, Harris LN, Ryals RH, "Examination of the antiglycemic properties of vinegar in healthy adults," *Annals of Nutrition Metabolism*, 2010;56(1):74-9. doi: 10.1159/000272133

"Keep the Nutrients," *Food Thinkers*.
http://storypages.foodthinkers.com/keep-the-nutrients/

Knapton, S, "Fasting for three days can regenerate entire immune system, study finds," *The Telegraph*, Telegraph Media Group. 5 June 2014. http://www.telegraph.co.uk/news/uknews/10878625/Fasting-for-three-days-can-regenerate-entire-immune-system-study-finds.html

Kondo T, Kishi M, Fushimi T, Kaga T, "Acetic acid upregulates the expression of genes for fatty acid oxidation enzymes in liver to suppress body fat accumulation," *Journal of Agriculture and Food Chemistry*, 2009 Jul 8;57(13):5982-6. doi: 10.1021/jf900470c

Kondo T, Kishi M, Fushimi T, Ugajin S, Kaga T, "Vinegar intake reduces body weight, body fat mass, and serum triglyceride levels in obese Japanese subjects." *Bioscience, Biotechnology, and Biochemistry,* 2009 Aug;73 (8):1837-43. Epub 2009 Aug 7.

Kondo S, Tayama K, Tsukamoto Y, Ikeda K, Yamori Y, "Antihypertensive effects of acetic acid and vinegar on spontaneously hypertensive rats," *Bioscience, Biotechnology, and Biochemistry,* 2001 Dec;65(12):2690-4.

Leeman M, Ostman E, Björck I, "Vinegar dressing and cold storage of potatoes lowers postprandial glycaemic and insulinaemic responses in healthy subjects," *European Journal of Clinical Nutrition.* 2005 Nov;59(11):1266-71.

Lehman, S, "Is Decaf Green Tea as Healthy as Regular Green Tea?" *About Health.* About.com, 17 Feb 2016 http://nutrition.about.com/od/askyournutritionist/f/decafgreen.htm

Liljeberg H, Björck I, "Delayed gastric emptying rate may explain improved glycaemia in healthy subjects to a starchy meal with added vinegar," *European Journal of Clinical Nutrition,* 1998 May;52(5):368-71.

Liska, DJ, "The Detoxification Enzyme System," *Alternative Medicine Review*, Thorne Research, Inc. 1998; 3(3)187. PDF e-book.

Maki KC, Pelkman CL, Finocchiaro ET, Kelley KM, Lawless AL, Schild AL, Rains TM, "Resistant starch from high-amylose maize increases insulin sensitivity in overweight and obese men," *J Nutr.* 2012 Apr;142(4):717-23. doi: 10.3945/jn.111.152975. Epub 2012 Feb 22.

Mandel SA, Amit T, Weinreb O, Reznichenko L, Youdim MB, "Simultaneous manipulation of multiple brain targets by green tea catechins: a potential neuroprotective strategy for Alzheimer and Parkinson diseases," *CNS Neuroscience Therapy,* 2008 Winter;14(4):352-65. doi: 10.1111/j.1755-5949.2008.00060.x

"Mother Nature's All-In-One, All-Natural, Cure-All, and Multi-Purpose Life Elixir." The Alternative Daily. http://www.thealternativedaily.com/pages/acvspecial.php?AFFID=%20151114&subid=SLACV

Nathan PJ, Lu K, Gray M, Oliver C, "The neuropharmacology of L-theanine(N-ethyl-L-glutamine): a possible neuroprotective and cognitive enhancing agent," *Journal of Herbal Pharmacother.* 2006;6(2):21-30

Onwuka, GI, "Soaking, Boiling, and Antinutritional Factors in Pigeon Peas (Cajanus cajan) and Cowpeas (Vigna unguiculata)," *Journal of Food Processing and Preservation,* 2006; 30(5): 616-630, doi: 10.1111/j.1745-4549.2006.00092.x

Ostman E, Granfeldt Y, Persson L, and Björck I, "Vinegar supplementation lowers glucose and insulin responses and increases satiety after a bread meal in healthy subjects," *European Journal of Clinical Nutrition.* 2005 Sep;59(9):983-8

Pizzutia D, Budaa A, D'Odoricoa A, D'Incàa R, Chiarellib S, Curionic A, Martinesa D, "Lack of intestinal mucosal toxicity of *Triticum monococcum* in celiac disease patients," *Scandinavian Journal of Gastroenterology* 2006; 41(11): 1305-1311, doi: 10.1080/00365520600699983

"Protein." *Better Health Channel.* State of Victoria. https://www.betterhealth.vic.gov.au/health/healthyliving/protein

Rasyid A, Lelo A, "The effect of curcumin and placebo on human gall-bladder function: an ultrasound study," *Aliment Pharmacology Therapy.* 1999 Feb;13(2):245-9

Raynor DA, Phelan S, Hill JO, Wing RR, "Television viewing and long-term weight maintenance: results from the National Weight Control Registry," *Obesity (Silver Spring).* 2006 Oct;14(10):1816-24.

Roan, S, "Running on empty: the pros and cons of fasting," *Los Angeles Times,* Los Angeles Times. 2 Feb 2009 http://articles.latimes.com/2009/feb/02/health/he-fasting2

Rosengren A, Wilhelmsen L, "Physical activity protects against coronary death and deaths from all causes in middle-aged men. Evidence from a 20-year follow-up of the primary prevention study in Göteborg," *Annals of Epidemiology,* 1997 Jan;7(1):69-75.

Rubio-Tapia A, Kyle R, Kaplan E, Johnson D, Page W, Erdtmann F, Brantner T, Kim W, Phelps T, Lahr B, Zinsmeister A, Melton L, Murray J, "Increased Prevalence and Mortality in Undiagnosed Celiac Disease," *Gastroenterology,* 2009; 137(1): 88-93 doi: 10.1053/j.gastro.2009.03.059

Rubio-Tapia A, Ludvigsson J, Brantner T, Murray J, Everhart J, "The Prevalence of Celiac Disease in the United States," *American Journal of Gastroenterology* 2012; 107:1538-1544; doi:10.1038/ajg.2012.219

Rutala WA, Barbee SL, Aguiar NC, Sobsey MD, Weber DJ, "Antimicrobial activity of home disinfectants and natural products against potential human pathogens," *Infect Control Hosp Epidemiology,* 2000 Jan;21(1):33-8

Sarsan A, Ardiç F, Ozgen M, Topuz O, Sermez Y, "The effects of aerobic and resistance exercises in obese women," *Clinical Rehabilitation.* 2006 Sep;20(9):773-82.

Seki T, Morimura S, Shigematsu T, Maeda H, Kida K, "Antitumor activity of rice-shochu post-distillation slurry and vinegar produced from the post-distillation slurry via oral administration in a mouse model," *Biofactors.* 2004;22(1-4):103-5.

Sekirov I, Russell S, Antunes L, Finlay B, "Gut Microbiota in Health and Disease," *Physiological Reviews,* 2010; 90(3): 859-904 doi: 10.1152/physrev.00045.2009

Shimoji Y, Kohno H, Nanda K, Nishikawa Y, Ohigashi H, Uenakai K, Tanaka T, "Extract of Kurosu, a vinegar from unpolished rice, inhibits azoxymethane-induced colon carcinogenesis in male F344 rats," *Nutrition Cancer.* 2004;49(2):170-3

Shishehbor F, Mansoori A, Sarkaki AR, Jalali MT, S.M. Latifi SM. "Apple Cider Vinegar Attenuates Lipid Profile in Normal and Diabetic Rats." Pakistan Journal of Biological Sciences. 11(23):2634-2638, 2008.

Shomon, M, "Sleep More, Lose Weight," *About Health.* About.com. 15 Dec 2014. http://thyroid.about .com/od/loseweightsuccessfully/a/sleepdiet.htm

Smith, R, "Sleeping for More Than Nine Hours May Help Weight Loss: Research," *The Telegraph.* Telegraph Media Group. 1 May 2012. http://www.telegraph.co.uk/news/health/news/9236158/ Sleeping-for-more-than-nine-hours-may-help-weight-loss-research.html

St-Onge MP, Roberts A, Chen J, Kelleman M, O'Keeffe M, RoyChoudhury A, Jones P, "Short sleep duration increases energy intakes but does not change energy expenditure in normal-weight individuals," *American Journal of Clinical Nutrition,* 29 June 2011. doi: 10.3945/ajcn.111.013904.

Stanway, P, "An Apple a Day Keeps the Doctor Away . . . And Prevents Asthma and Beats Hiccups!" *The Daily Mail,* Associated Newspapers, Ltd. 19 April 2011. http://www.dailymail.co.uk/health/ article-1378303/An-apple-day-keeps-doctor-away--And-prevents-asthma-beats-hiccups. html

Troncone R, Jabri B, "Coeliac Disease and Gluten Sensitivity," *Journal of Internal Medicine.* 269, no: 6 (2011): 582-590, doi: 10.1111/j.1365-2796.2011.02385.x

Van Walleghen EL, Orr JS, Gentile CL, Davy BM, "Pre-meal water consumption reduces meal energy intake in older but not younger subjects," *Obesity (Silver Spring).* 2007 Jan;15(1):93-9.

Vilppula A, Collin P, Mäki M, Valve R, Luostarinen M, Krekelä I, Patrikainen H, Kaukinen K, Luostarinen L, "Undetected coeliac disease in the elderly: a biopsy-proven population-based study," *Dig Liver Dis.* 2008 Oct;40(10):809-13. doi: 10.1016/j.dld.2008.03.013. Epub 2008 May 7.

Wakim-Fleming, J, "Celiac Disease and Malabsorptive Disorders," *Cleveland Clinic*, The Cleveland Clinic Foundation. Oct 2012. http://www.clevelandclinicmeded.com/medicalpubs/ diseasemanagement/gastroenterology/celiac-disease-malabsorptive-disorders/

"Weed Control the Natural Way." The Dirt Doctor. https://www.dirtdoctor.com/garden/Weed-Control-Natural-Way_vq340.htm

White A, Johnston C, "Vinegar Ingestion at Bedtime Moderates Waking Glucose Concentrations in Adults With Well-Controlled Type 2 Diabetes," *American Diabetes Association.* American Diabetes Association. 30 November 2014. http://care.diabetesjournals.org/content/30/11/ 2814.ful

"Why You Should Be Drinking Peppermint Herb Tea Before Bed," *Fit Day*, Internet Brands, Inc. http://www.fitday.com/fitness-articles/nutrition/healthy-eating/why-you-should-be-drinking-peppermint-herb-tea-before-bed.html

Wing RR, Phelan S, "Long-term weight loss maintenance," *American Journal of Clinical Nutrition*, 2005 Jul;82(1 Suppl):222S-225S.

Wong, CND, "Apple Cider Vinegar for Weight Loss: Can It Help You Shed Pounds?" *Alternative Medicine*. About. http://altmedicine.about.com/od/applecidervinegardiet/a/Apple-Cider-Vinegar-Weight-Loss.htm

Wu CW, Chen YC, Yu L, Chen HI, Jen CJ, Huang AM, Tsai HJ, Chang YT, Kuo YM, "Treadmill exercise counteracts the suppressive effects of peripheral lipopolysaccharide on hippocampal neurogenesis and learning and memory," *Journal of Neurochem*. 2007 Dec;103(6):2471-81. Epub 2007 Oct 22.

Yuan JH, Li YQ, Yang XY, " Inhibition of Epigallocatechin Gallate on Orthotropic Colon Cancer by Upregulating the Nrf2-UGT1A Signal Pathway in Nude Mice," *Pharmacology*, 2007;80:269-278, doi: 10.1159/000106447

Yu-Xiao Y, Lewis J, Epstein S, Metz D, "Long-term Proton Pump Inhibitor Therapy and Risk of Hip Fracture," *JAMA*. 2006;296(24):2947-2953. doi:10.1001/jama.296.24.2947

Zafar, J, "Apple Cider Vinegar: The Wonder 'Drug' of Yesterday and Today," *Food Matters*. Food Matters International Pty Ltd. 8 April 2011. http://www.foodmatters.tv/articles-1/apple-cider-vinegar-the-wonder-drug-of-yesterday-and-today

Index